4 Frontiers in European Radiology

Editors-in-Chief

A. L. Baert · E. Boijsen
W. A. Fuchs · F. H.W. Heuck

Springer-Verlag
Berlin Heidelberg New York Tokyo 1984

Professor Dr. Albert L. Baert
Universitaire Ziekenhuizen, Department of Diagnostic Radiology,
Capucijnenvoer 35, B-3000 Leuven

Professor Dr. Erik Boijsen
University Hospital, Department of Diagnostic Radiology, S-22185 Lund

Professor Dr. Walter A. Fuchs
Inselspital Bern, Institut für Diagnostische Radiologie der Universität,
CH-3010 Bern

Professor Dr. Friedrich H. W. Heuck
Radiologisches Institut im Zentrum Radiologie, Katharinenhospital
(Lehrkrankenhaus der Universität Tübingen),
Kriegsbergstr. 60, D-7000 Stuttgart

With 82 Figures (in 144 Separate Illustrations)

ISBN-13: 978-3-642-69719-7 e-ISBN-13: 978-3-642-69717-3
DOI: 10.1007/978-3-642-69717-3

2121/3130-543210

Contents

Therapeutic Angiography in Neuroradiology: Clinical Objectives and Results

P. Lasjaunias, P. Halimi, and L. Lopez-Ibor[1]

1 Introduction

Embolization procedures now dominate therapeutic angiography. Although not presented in this review, chemotherapy by infusion in situ, chemoembolization by microspheres, and angioplasty should not be forgotten.

Following *Djindjian*'s first embolizations, several teams in France and in other countries have spent more than 10 years developing new concepts, new methods, and new equipment. The rapidity of evolution requires consideration of embolization technique at a conceptual level.

Historically, two major factors have led to improvement in embolization procedures:

1. Increasing knowledge of the radioanatomy of the arteries of head and neck down to a caliber of 200–300 μm, regardless of the vascular arrangement (*Lasjaunias* 1981).
2. The development of new catheters and embolic agents allowing embolization of the lesional nidus itself (*Berenstein* and *Kricheff* 1979a, b; *Berenstein* 1980; *Berenstein* and *Kricheff* 1981; *Kerber* et al. 1979; *Kunstlinger* et al. 1981; *Vinters* et al. 1981).

The immediate consequences of these two advances are safety and reliability of the procedures and clinical efficiency. In 10 years, we have progressed from en-

1 Service de Radiologie, Hôpital Bicêtre, Université Paris XI, 78, Rue du Général Leclerc, F-94 270 Kremlin-Bicêtre. Submitted for publication in March 1983

dovascular arterial ligation with strips of Gelfoam and balls of Silastic to microscopic arterial occlusion within the target, with no possibility of collateral circulation. Precise topographical diagnosis gives exact information on the composition of any lesion, therefore enabling selection of the best arterial route to the nidus.

The neuroradiologist becomes the user of the diagnostic imaging facilities, which must provide the necessary information for selection of the best approach. Global vascular explorations, although providing the diagnosis in most situations, do not allow appreciation of the feasibility of embolization in a given patient. Proper arterial mapping with superselective analysis is therefore mandatory.

In general, it is often easier to treat a post-traumatic vascular problem, as the vascular system is healthy and its behavior predictable. In contrast, the response of the vascular system is rarely predictable in congenital arteriovenous malformations (AVMs) or hereditary conditions (e.g., Rendu-Osler-Weber disease) – with or without angiogenetic activity. This is illustrated perfectly by the endovascular treatment of traumatic and spontaneous caroticocavernous fistulas: most traumatic cases can be treated successfully, but spontaneous cases are more difficult to heal completely (*Berenstein* et al. 1980; *Debrun* et al. 1981 a; *Picard* et al. 1974 a.).

It seems that vascular damage after trauma only needs assistance in returning to normal; even a simple proximal embolization may bring the reward of excellent results. Endovascular treatment of "diseases", however, requires microembolization (fluid agent or microparticles) to produce a stable clinical result.

Judgment of the result of embolization cannot rest merely on the angiographic appearance of the occlusion; clinical signs must be considered. This obliges the neuroradiologist to follow up patients clinically in order to assess the results, being the only person to know the patient's condition before treatment and what has been achieved during embolization.

The nature and frequency of complications has changed with modern developments in technique. Details will not be discussed here, but it should be remembered that in a cooperative study in 1978, *Doyon* et al. showed that 85% of embolization complications in the head, neck, and spinal areas resulted from inappropriate personal decisions taken during the procedure. This emphasizes the need for thorough training of angiographers, perfect knowledge of vascular anatomy, familiarity with the effect and manipulation of different embolic agents, good clinical background in the diseases of these areas, and close cooperation with the appropriate diagnostic or therapeutic specialists.

2 Applications

2.1 Hemorrhage

Embolization presents an alternative to surgical ligation, the results of which are generally controversial and unreliable (*Merland* et al. 1981). In the head and neck, emergency surgical ligation is frequently blind and therefore imprecise; far from the site of hemorrhage, ligation often does not even close the artery which is bleeding, but a proximal trunk, and collateral circulation can develop almost instantaneously. This approach always ignores the possibility of anatomical variants.

In contrast, superselective angiography and embolization can achieve distal occlusion, and sometimes identification of the site of bleeding enables specific hemostasis. In all situations, whatever the vascular pattern, the symptomatic area can be reached.

Hemorrhages can occur:

1. Spontaneously: in certain angiomatoses (Rendu-Osler-Weber) and tumors (juvenile angiofibroma), in coagulation factor deficiencies, in arterial ulceration (cancer spread sequelae of radiotherapy), and in AVMs (dural, cerebral, oral, etc.).
2. Following trauma: complex maxillofacial fractures can be responsible for uncontrollable epistaxis, or a preexisting AVM can rupture, perhaps triggered by such minimal trauma as may occur on eating or on brushing of the teeth.
3. At operation: during surgery for removal of an hypervascularized lesion, or when the presence of the lesion is unsuspected (e.g., tooth extraction and mandibular AVM).

In the embolization of hemorrhages, emphasis is laid on three points:

1. The stability of the hemostasis. This depends on the stabilization of the disease itself, on how distal the occlusion is, and on the type of embolic agent (resorbable or not).
2. Prophylactic treatment in lesions which threaten to bleed.
3. Embolization in emergency situations. A competent angiographic team and reliable well-maintained radiological equipment must be available 24 hours a day. Embolization sometimes remains hard to perform when the target is difficult to reach because of regional arterial collapse, spasm, nasal packing (epistaxis) or arterial changes after radiotherapy.

Taking epistaxis as an example, it should be remembered that the symptoms are more important than the angiographic appearance (Fig. 1). The latter is normal in some massive epistaxis requiring embolization, and in other cases the nasal mucosae opacification can appear almost abnormal without symptom, therefore without need for treatment.

2.2 Tumor Mass

Embolization reduces the tumor mass in situations where enlargement of the tumor has been rapid or where its hypervascular or cavernous nature is important (*Lasjaunias* and *Doyon* 1980; *Lasjaunias* et al. 1980). The result is improvement in the clinical symptoms related to tumor mass. Examples of such clinical situations are:

- Swallowing disorders in tumors of the tongue or pharynx
- Respiratory disorders caused by choanal obstruction (*Lasjaunias* et al. 1980)
- Cosmetic problems (*Tazi* et al. 1981)
- Functional disorders in lesions of the oral cavity which impair bilabial or occlusal contact and therefore mandibular growth (*Fellus* et al. 1979)
- Disorders in osseous growth following local hyperemia with bony dysmorphism and hypertrophy
- Giant aneurysms (Fig. 2) (*Debrun* et al. 1981 b)

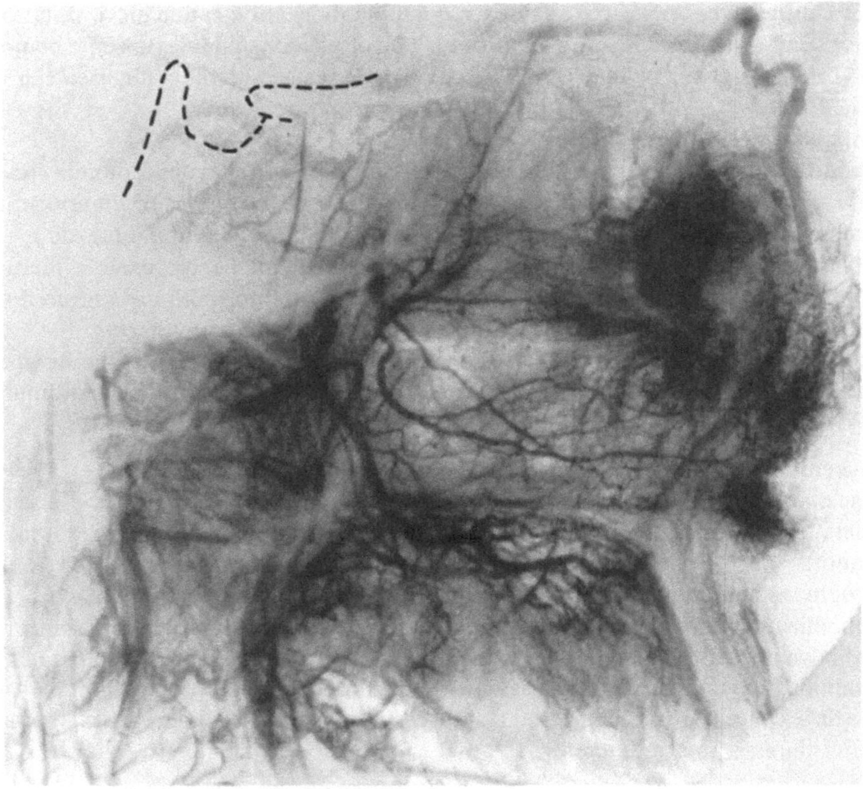

a

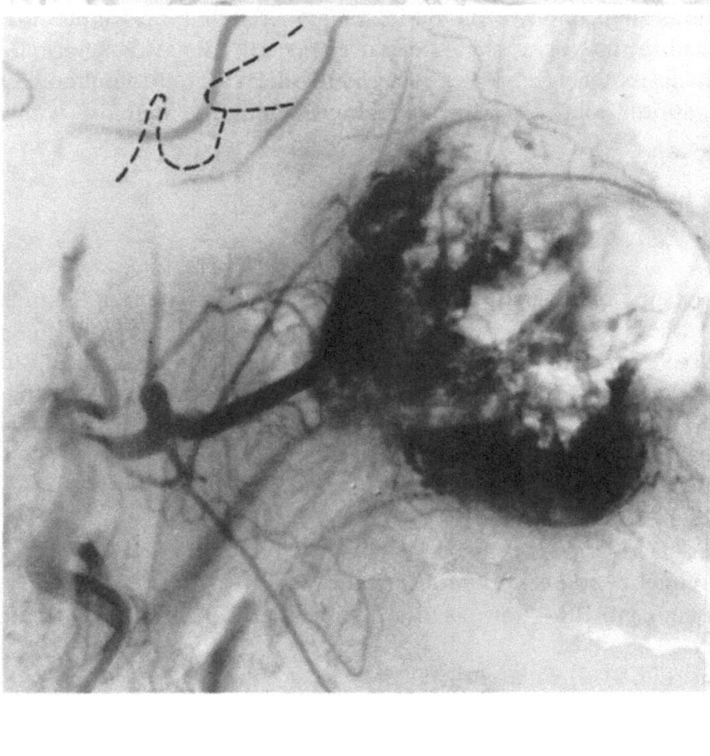

b

Fig. 1a, b

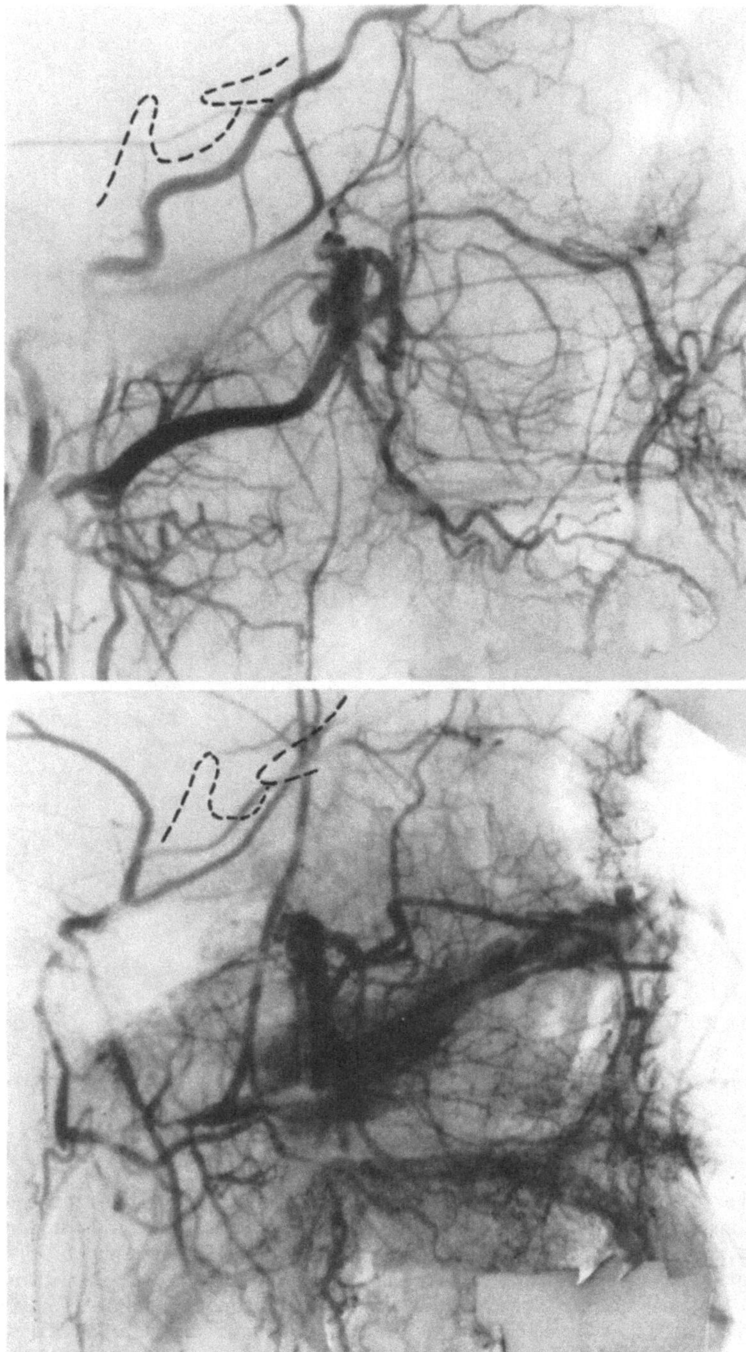

c

d

Fig. 1 c, d

Legend see page 6

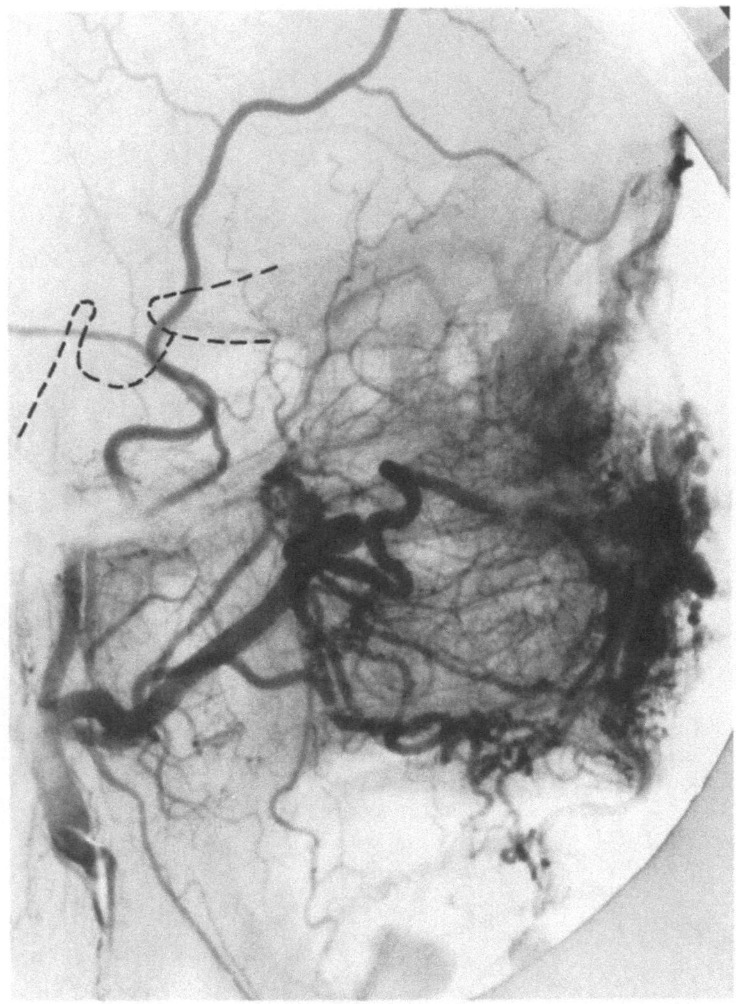

Fig. 1e

Fig. 1a–g. Angiograms after distal external carotid injections, demonstrating the absence of relationship between the intensity of nasal mucosae opacification and the importance of clinical symptoms. **a** 30-year-old female with no maxillofacial symptoms. **b** 50-year-old male, epistaxis with maxillary sinus metastasis. **c** Intense ipsilateral epistaxis with major maxillofacial trauma requiring blood transfusions. **d** Spontaneous epistaxis in a 50-year-old female with no personal or familial history of bleeding; blood transfusions. **e** Vascular malformations of the nasal fossa (inferior turbinate and alar region) with no bleeding. **f, g** two cases (from different families) of Rendu-Osler-Weber disease in a 35-year-old female (**f**) and a 50-year-old male (**g**), both presenting intense epistaxis requiring blood transfusion. Cases **b–g** were successfully embolized for hemostasis. Case **e** was also embolized before surgery, with an immediate satisfactory effect on the bleeding (*Lasjaunias* 1983)

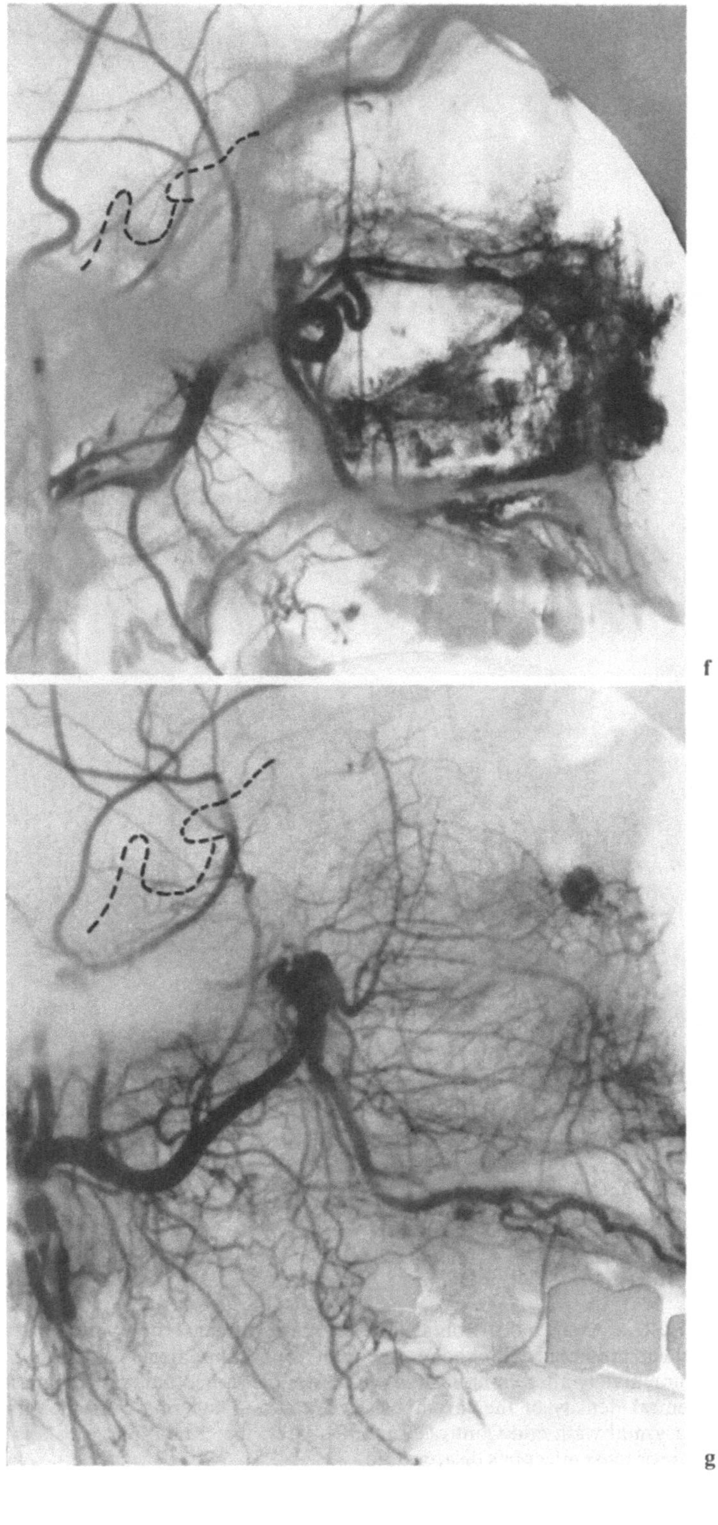

Fig. 1 f, g

a, b

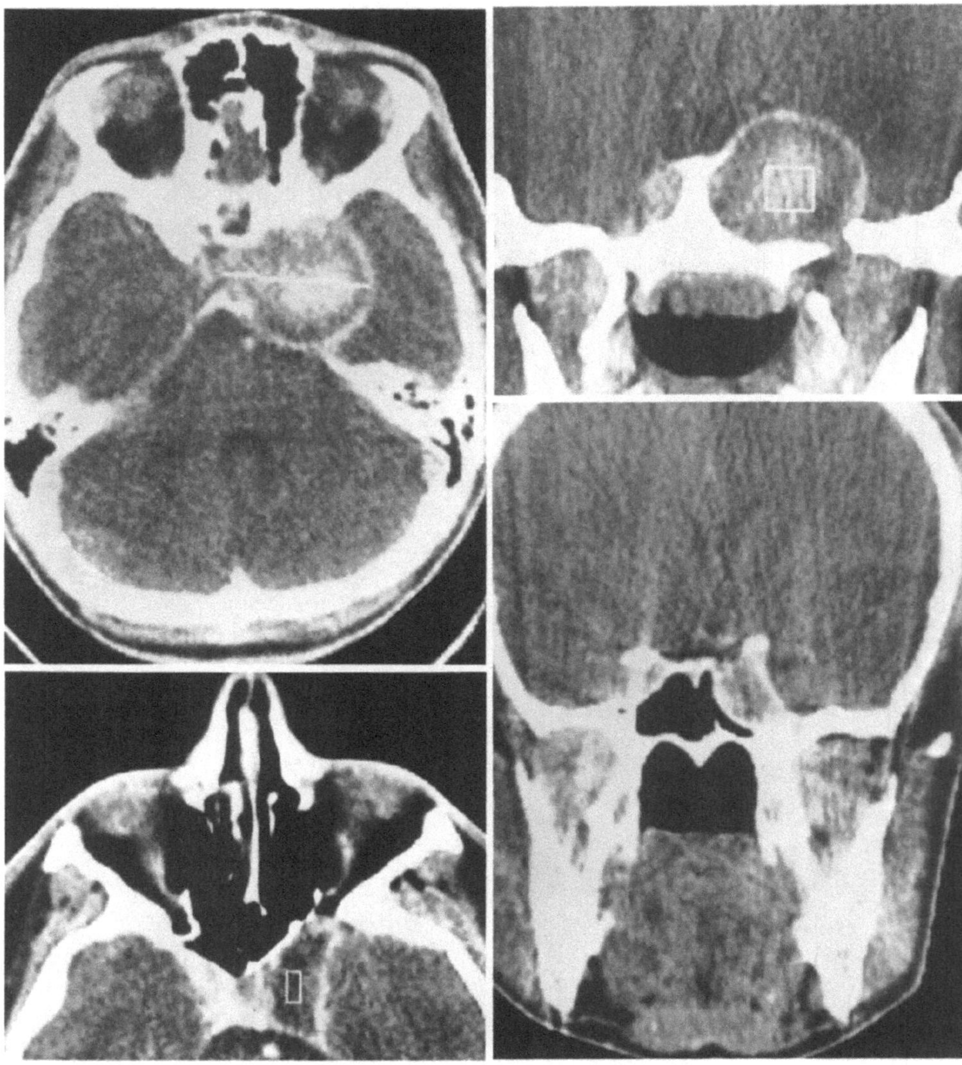

c, d

Fig. 2. a Axial and **b** frontal CT of a giant intracavernous internal carotid artery aneurysm, which presented with sudden complete ophthalmoplegia and fifth cranial nerve anesthesia, immediately after embolization with a double-lumen balloon catheter and thrombin. Note the central density of the thrombosis induced and the ring corresponding to the enhanced aneurysmal wall. **c, d** Controls 9 months later: the cranial nerve palsies have regressed and the tumor mass effect has disappeared

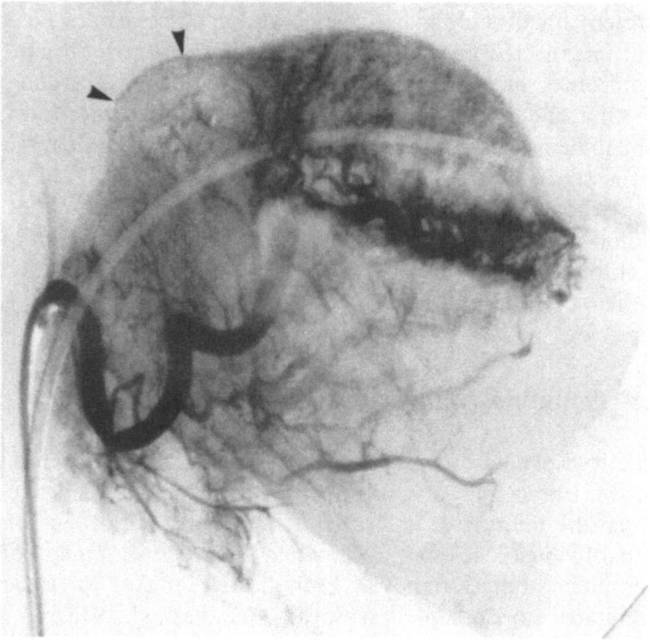

Fig. 3. Selective injection of the lingual artery in a case of painful cavernous hemangioma (*arrowheads*). The pain and tumor mass effect disappeared clinically after embolization (PVA 500–1000 μm) so no surgery has been performed

Paradoxically, an AVM with a predominant cellular component can respond better to embolization than a purely vascular malformation with a large vascular component. The changes brought about by embolization are not immediate, tumor reduction progressing slowly until a new equilibrium is reached (e.g., in tongue hemolymphangiomas) (*Lasjaunias* and *Doyon* 1980). In highly vascular lesions, embolization must be complete if it is to achieve a significant reduction in mass, whereas incomplete embolization can be effective in highly cellular tumors, the only condition being that the emboli must reach the tumor bed.

The decision whether to perform complete or uncomplete, staged or immediate embolization depends on intralesional vascular pattern, i.e., single or multiple compartments (*Lasjaunias* 1983; *Moret* et al. 1980). This type of analysis enables design of an individual tailored strategy in every patient, which is particularly beneficial in difficult cases.

2.3 Pain

Pain related to tumor mass will naturally be alleviated if the mass is reduced. Some types of pain (e.g., vertebral angioma) are of vascular origin and their mechanism is hardly understood, but the effect of embolization is often spectacular (Fig. 3). Pain relief is not always achieved in cancer, but can be obtained in most cases. At the present time, neuralgias (trigeminal, hypoglossal) are not treated by embolization, but unexpected anesthesias in cranial nerve territories and alleviation of neuralgic syndromes have been observed following embolization (*Lasjaunias* and *Doyon* 1980; *Lasjaunias* et al. 1981). The mechanisms are poorly understood, and steal phenomena close to hypervascularized tumors (e.g., paraganglioma) are sometimes discussed.

Headaches intractable to medical treatment sometimes disappear after embolization of the middle meningeal artery, unfortunately with no reliable angiographic pictures. This has also been observed during embolization of the sole dural component of a cerebral AVM.

2.4 Evolution, Malignancy, and Recurrence

The role played by embolization in the decrease in tumor recurrence is difficult to prove. Embolization is still possible in recurrent benign lesions (e.g., meningioma) when the recurrence is located at the vascular entrance of the original tumor, and can obviously be employed when the redevelopment of the tumor follows incomplete surgical removal. Embolization makes for easier surgery and therefore facilitates more complete removal (*Manelfe* et al. 1978).

Comparisons of series in cooperative studies of presurgical embolization unfortunately contain two human variables, the skills of the angiographers and of the surgeons, and fail to assess the technique itself. Personal series, although smaller, are sometimes more significant in that they illustrate the results of homogeneous approach.

With regard to evolution of malignant lesions or secondary transformation of benign tumors, chemoembolization using spheres loaded with chemotoxins should give good results in the near future (*Madoule* et al. 1981).

Angiogenetic factors are though to be involved in some malignant developments (e.g., glioblastomas) (*Brem* 1976). One can theorize that disarterialization by means of embolization in this situation would limit the angiogenic effect of a tumor and stabilize its development. One should, however, embolize the healthy tissues in the neighborhood of a tumor to prevent its extension.

Some lesions evolve with the menstrual cycle (growing in the second half of the cycle), or with pregnancy (growing during the last trimester): meningiomas, neurinomas, cavernous hemangiomas, hemolymphangiomas, some telangiectasias (e.g., Rendu-Osler-Weber disease). Empirically, embolization stabilizes the lesions with periodic evolution and generally any lesion which clinically follows hormonal changes. Some of them present specific receptors to sexual hormones or steroids; however, no satisfactory explanation for the successes and failures of embolization or for the periodic swelling has been given. Similarly, acute swelling of head and neck AVMs in prepubertal children following infections and dental eruptions subsides after distal embolization (*Lasjaunias* and *Doyon* 1981).

2.5 Vascular Bruits

Vascular bruits are often due to the hyperpulsatility of a vessel in contact with the base of the skull, particularly the temporal bone, or to the turbulence within such a vessel. Embolization realizing an occlusion in situ can make this symptom disappear, but the effect on the symptom will depend on the effect on the responsible disease (AVM, tumor with arteriovenous fistula).

Vascular bruits are often associated with venous hyperpressure, and the clinical presentation will then depend on the vein involved (cavernous sinus, ophthalmic vein, cerebral vein, spinal vein, etc.) and the territory it drains.

2.6 Secreting Lesions

Some tumors of head and neck have primitive secreting activities (parathyroid adenomas, paragangliomas, etc.); some of them are metastatic. Embolization (pure or with contrast infusion) has a good effect on this type of lesion. The cell differentiation evidenced by the secreting activity tolerates ischemia poorly. The stabilization of the effect obtained will depend on the quantity of tissue destroyed; complete embolization is mandatory for a definitive and stable result. Contrast infusion alone is often sufficient to obtain a stable cure if the selectivity achieved is close enough to the tumor.

2.7 Some Specific Neuroradiological Lesions

2.7.1 Juvenile Angiofibroma

Juvenile angiofibromas (Fig. 4) (*Djindjian* and *Merland* 1978; *Lasjaunias* et al. 1980; *Manelfe* et al. 1978; *Riche* et al. 1979) develop in the cavum and constitute the most typical benign surgical tumor: young male patient, tumor hypervascularized, surgical, highly hemorrhagic, infiltrating and destructive, producing choanal occlusion. Malignant transformation is only rarely observed, and then only after radiotherapy. Recurrence is usually a sequel of incomplete surgery. The main danger is represented by recurrence and by intracranial extension.

Embolization in this disease has several objectives (e.g., reduction of tumor mass, alleviation of hemorrhage), and continues to be used presurgically by most french teams. It improves surgical results: less than 10% recurrence, instead of 30%–50% without embolization.

The most appropriate embolic agents with regard to the angioarchitecture of these tumors are small particles of 250–400 μm polyvinyl alcohol foam (PVA) or dura mater. Smaller agents (particules or fluids) are dangerous (cranial nerves, carotid anastomoses), and bigger ones (balloons or Silastic balls, reproduce the ineffectiveness of proximal ligations.

Other lesions developing in the same area may also be affected by the embolization, whether or not they are accessible to surgery (e.g., papillomas, cancers, hemangiopericytomas, paragangliomas). In addition, embolization makes diagnostic biopsy safe.

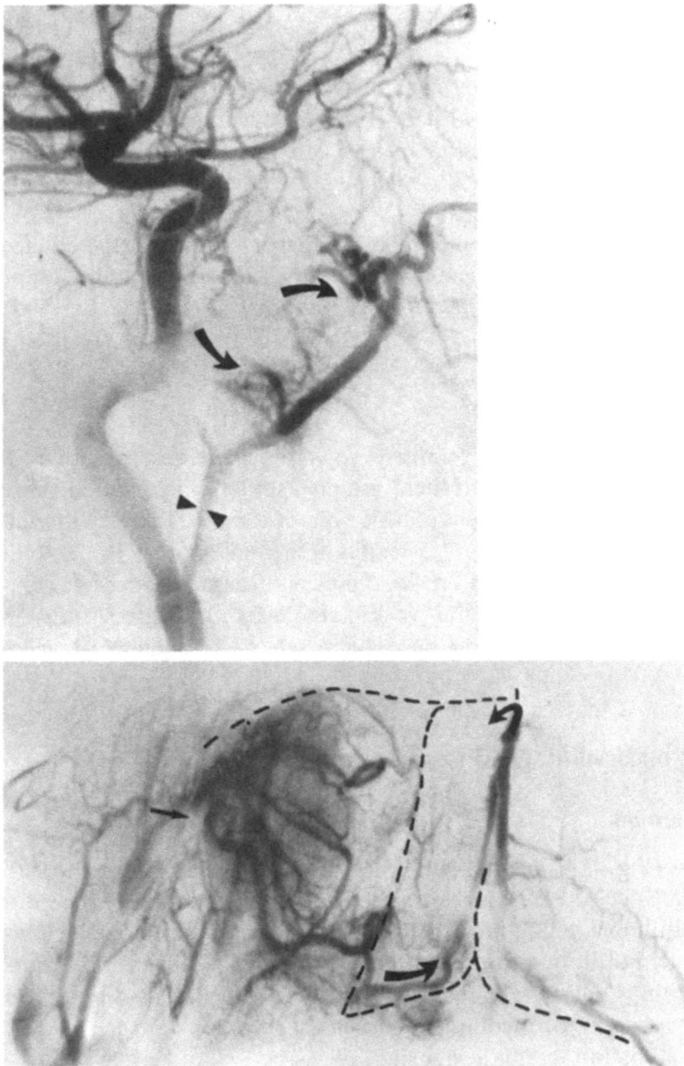
a

b

Fig. 4 a, b

Fig. 4. **a** Internal carotid injection in a case of bleeding juvenile angiofibroma. Internal maxillary ligation (*arrowheads*) has been carried out, but the internal carotid artery siphon through the foramen rotundum and ovale (*curved arrows*) reconstitutes the distal internal maxillary artery. **b** Selective injection of the distal anterior division of the ascending pharyngeal artery (*arrow*). Note the permeable soft palate anastomosis (*curved arrow*) which allows access to the internal maxillary from below (*curved arrow*). **c** Control during embolization (isobutyl). Note the defects in embolization (*open arrows*). The anastomosis (*curved arrow*) is still open. **d** Final control angiography of the internal carotid artery. No supply to the cavum, no collateral circulation visible. Embolization has been achieved exclusively through the palatine system (*Lasjaunias* 1983)

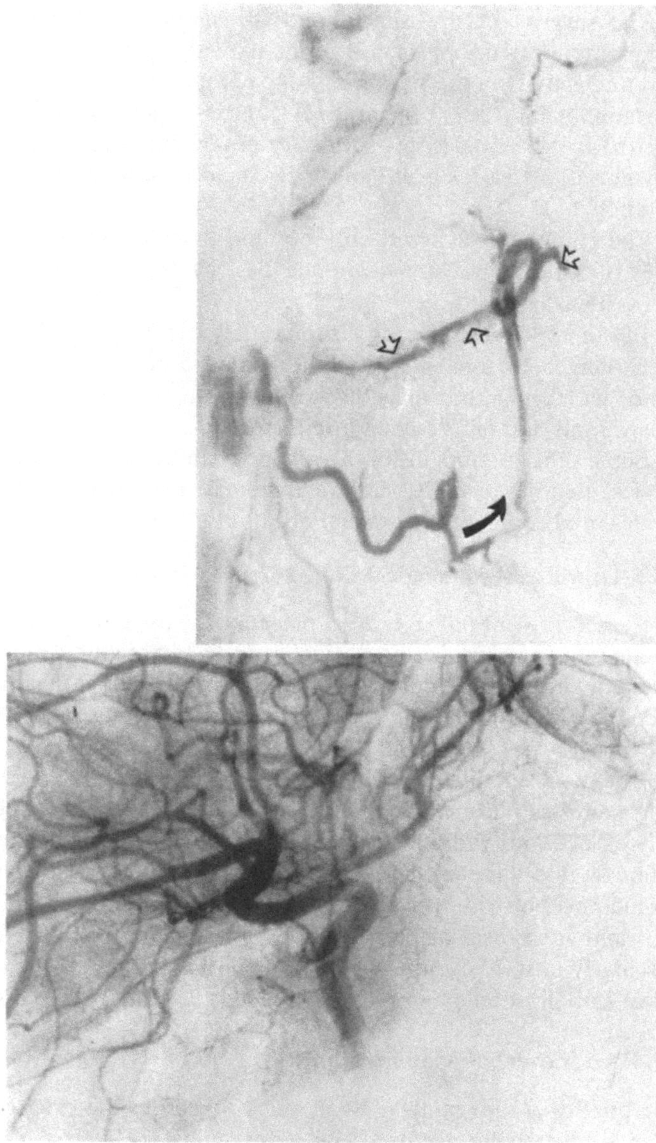

c

Fig. 4 c, d

d

2.7.2 Paraganglioma

Tympanic, jugular, vagal, or carotid, paragangliomas all present common properties: highly vascularized, sometimes multifocal (10%), slowly increasing in size, constantly supplied by the ascending pharyngeal artery (*Djindjian* and *Merland* 1978; *Lasjaunias* 1983; *Lasjaunias* et al. 1981; *Manelfe* et al. 1978; *Moret* et al. 1980). The clinical presentation reflects tumor mass, effect on cranial nerves, bone destruction, arterial steal, hormonal secretion (catecholamines, serotonin), and arteriovenous shunt.

The severity of the tumors and the surgical challenge depend on the cerebellopontine extension, the age of the patient, the internal carotid involvement, the secreting activity of the tumor, and the peroperative bleeding. The objectives of embolization will therefore be multiple: (a) presurgical to diminish peroperative bleeding; (b) if the lesion is not surgically removable, palliation by diminishing tumor mass, arterial steal or bruit, and the related neurological symptoms; (c) to combat secretion.

The embolic agents will only be fluid in exceptional unresectable lesions. Particles of 250–400 µm are again the best choice if there are no intratumoral arteriovenous fistulas.

In our experience of embolization in 30 cases from 1977 to 1982, we have never been obliged to use anything other than particles. The close relationship of the tumor with dangerous anastomoses always demands perfect knowledge of the arterial supply and of its angiographic aspects.

Some other tumors in this area which can be diagnosed during angiography are cervical neurinomas (IX, X), meningiomas, and hemangiomas. They are a priori surgical and can benefit from embolization.

2.7.3 Otorhinolaryngological Cancer

There is at present only a limited place for the use of endovascular techniques in the treatment of otorhinolaryngological cancers, but the indications should be extended. Antalgia and reduction in volume can be obtained, and these effects should be more widely known. Embolization in such tumors is a conservative treatment rather than one of last resort (*Manelfe* et al. 1978).

The most suitable materials are still dura mater or PVA of 400–800 µm. Resorbable agents should be avoided: it is difficult to catheterize cancerous vessels repeatedly as previous radiotherapy makes them hyperfragile. The objective of embolization should therefore be reached at the first attempt, if at all possible. The effect should never be widespread, but limited to one or a few specific locations.

Fluid substances or particles of below 250 µm must be avoided; these areas are vascularly unstable, and even when angiography has shown hypervascularity, nondistal embolization may result, producing a large and unnecessary necrosis.

2.7.4 Arteriovenous Malformations

The quality of the results now obtained illustrates the progress in techniques, catheters, and embolic agents. Four groups must be differentiated: (a) maxillofacial AVMs (*Djindjian* and *Merland* 1978; *Lasjaunias* and *Doyon* 1980, 1981; *Picard* et al. 1978; *Tazi* et al. 1981), (b) maxillofacial angiomatosis (*Lasjaunias* 1983; *Picard* et al. 1974b), (c) dural AVMs (*Lasjaunias* 1983; *Picard* et al. 1974a), and (d) intracranial (*Debrun* et al. 1978, 1982; *Epstein* and *Berenstein* 1981; *Luessenhop* and *Presber* 1975; *Serbinenko* 1974, 1978) and intradural spinal (*Merland* et al. 1980) AVMs.

2.7.4.1 Maxillofacial AVMs

The symptoms in maxillofacial AVMs (Fig. 5) consist of cosmetic problems (tumor mass effect, venous hypertension), neuralgias, hemorrhages, and functional disturbances (eyelids, tongue). Most complications, apart from the aggravation of these symptoms, are iatrogenic: antibodies after multiple transfusions, viral hepatitis, postirradiation malignant changes; in addition, multiple surgical ligations and excessively proximal embolization make the lesions untreatable transarterially.

In practice, embolization is indicated:
1. When the *entire* AVM can be surgically removed, whatever the symptoms
2. When the AVM involves serious *complications,* in which case the aim is only to treat the complication not to attempt a complete result; for example, in a stable and benign AVM with post-traumatic fistula, only the fistula should be treated
3. When other treatment close to the AVM is necessary (e.g., dental extraction with mandibular hemangioma) and presents a major risk of peroperative bleeding.

Relative contraindications to embolization are:
1. Angioma not requiring surgery where the only problem is a "moderate" cosmetic complaint. This is always difficult to assess and remains subjective and cultural.
2. A young subject without major symptoms. The prepubertal tendency to spontaneous favorable evolution should not be forgotten, and aggressive treatment must be prohibited.
3. Predominant cutaneous involvement. Embolization has no effect on a purely cutaneous lesion and the risk of necrosis is high.

The material to be used depends on the flow through the AVM and on the specific problems presented by the individual. In most cases particles are suitable exceptions being fistulas and large arteriovenous shunts, in which isobutyl has to be used with great care.

Embolization will often have to be done in two sittings; it is helpful to perform arterial mapping in a previous procedure. In this way, the material and protocol can best be adapted to the patient's specific problems.

These procedures are not universally agreed on. Some Anglo-Saxon teams, in particular, use only a fluid embolic agent (silicone) with flow control (*Berenstein* 1980). Their indications are broad, but some results are encouraging. Their experience is often limited, but is unique with this material.

The controversy over the choice of treatment highlights several difficulties in the therapeutic management of maxillofacial AVMs:

1. Angiographic and pathological classification do not help in the selection of therapy.
2. Each therapeutic experience is individual and nonreproducible.
3. Every lesion poses different clinical problems with different answers. The hardest symptoms to evaluate are cosmetic disorders, the psychological consequences of a given lesion depending on the patient's personality, social level, and environment, with the reactions of the doctor in charge also playing a part.
4. The morphological characteristics of an AVM are not predictive of its behavior. A highly evolutive lesion can have the same appearance as an inactive one.
5. Many aspects of hematolymphangiomas go unnoticed.

With regard to the pediatric population, almost all lesions have the potential of regressing before puberty. However, we feel that spontaneous regression may occur too late with regard to induced morphological disorders. A 30–45 min intervention

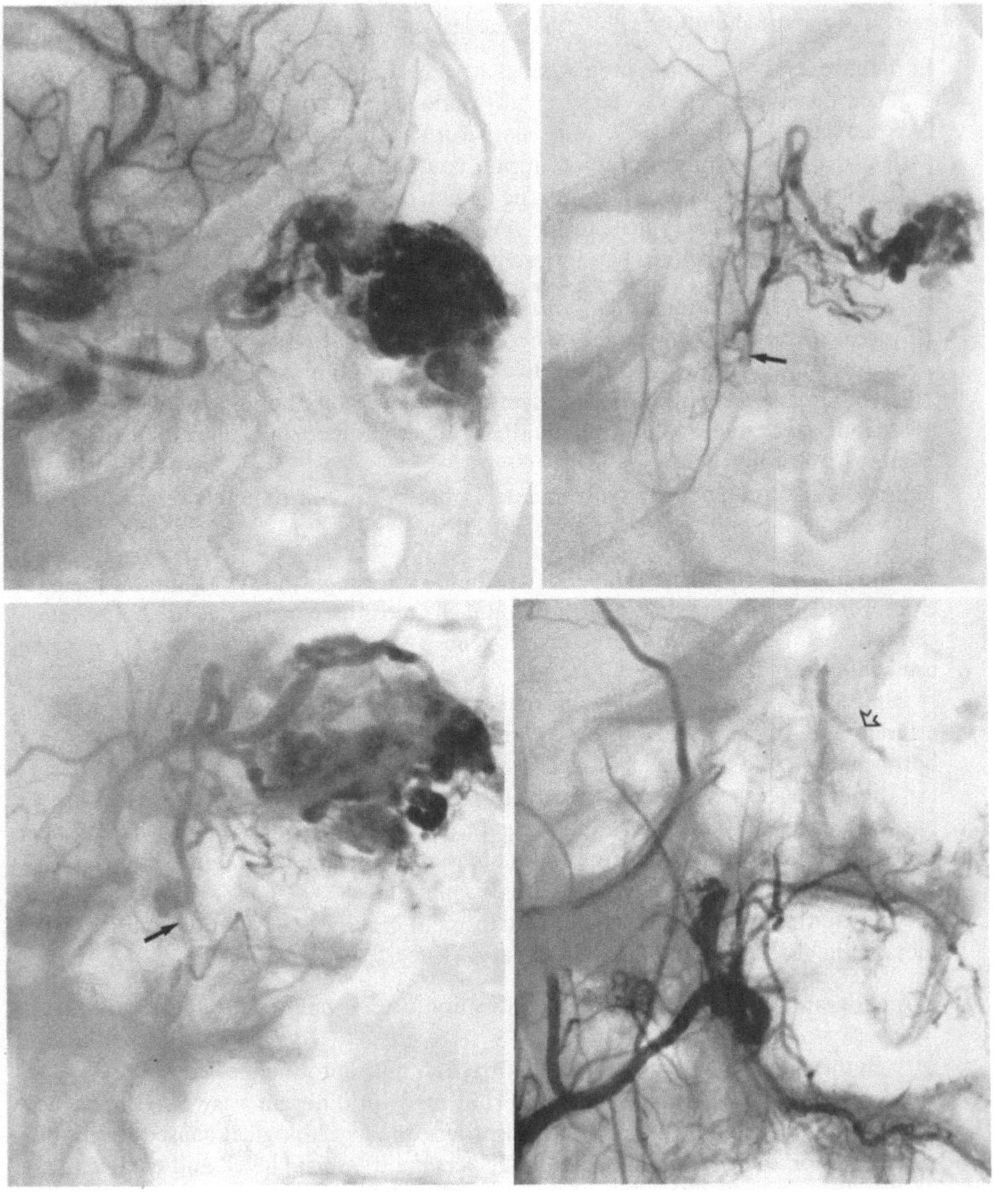

a, b

c, d

Fig. 5a–d

Fig. 5a–e. Bleeding palpebral AVM. **a** Internal carotid injection. **b, c** Lateral and oblique views the anterior deep temporal injection (*arrow*). Both systems fill the AVM, which can be considered as single-compartmented with two sources of supply. **d** Internal maxillary injection immediately after embolization of the anterior deep temporal artery alone with radiopaque isobutyl (*open arrow*). **e** Note, on the internal carotid injection following **d**, that the other feeder of the lesion is not longer functional, despite not being embolized

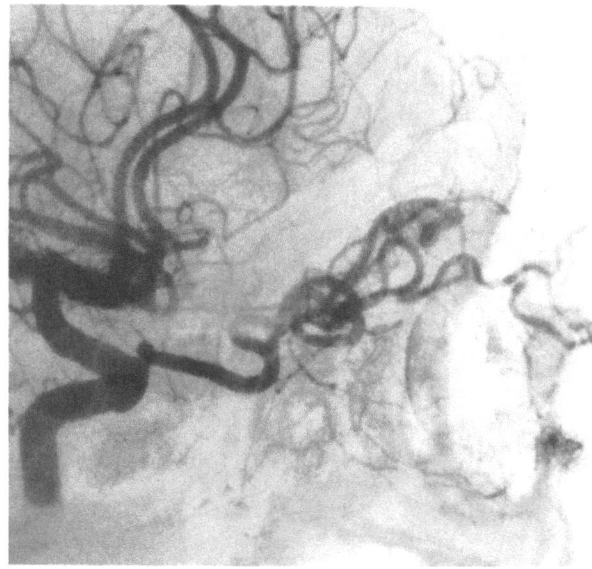

Fig. 5e

by a well-trained angiographer in a 2- to 4-year-old child is preferable to a reconstructive operation after 12 years of evolution, with the unpredictable surgical results and the psychological consequences of growing up with a maxillofacial AVM. However, we regard the following symptoms as indicating embolization: bleeding alteration of the maxillofacial growth, repeated acute swelling, pain, difficulties in respiration or swallowing, permanent ptosis in palpebral AVM.

2.7.4.2 Maxillofacial Angiomatosis

We will use Rendu-Osler-Weber disease as an example of angiomatosis. It is a dominant autosomal disease often revealed by epistaxis in adults. It is diffuse in location and can involve any tissue; however, major bleeding almost occur in the same regions (nasal cavities, digestive tract), other affected areas remaining almost asymptomatic (lips, gums, tongue, liver, skin).

The sole aims of embolization are to obtain hemostasis and prevent neurological complications (e.g., brain abscess with pulmonary arteriovenous fistula). Other types of treatment yield disappointing results and are often aggressive, compromising other approaches (e.g., ligation, radiotherapy).

Endovascular occlusion for epistaxis produces encouraging, though not very stable, results and never compromises any other approach. Therefore embolization should be carried out first and repeated unless angiography proves that the territory involved is or has become unreachable. The material to be used is again particles of 250–400 μm.

Preventive treatment in angiomas liable to bleed represents the ideal, but identification is not yet possible.

Widening of the vessel walls by means of intravenous administration of oestrogens has yielded good results. In situ delivery of these drugs using microspheres

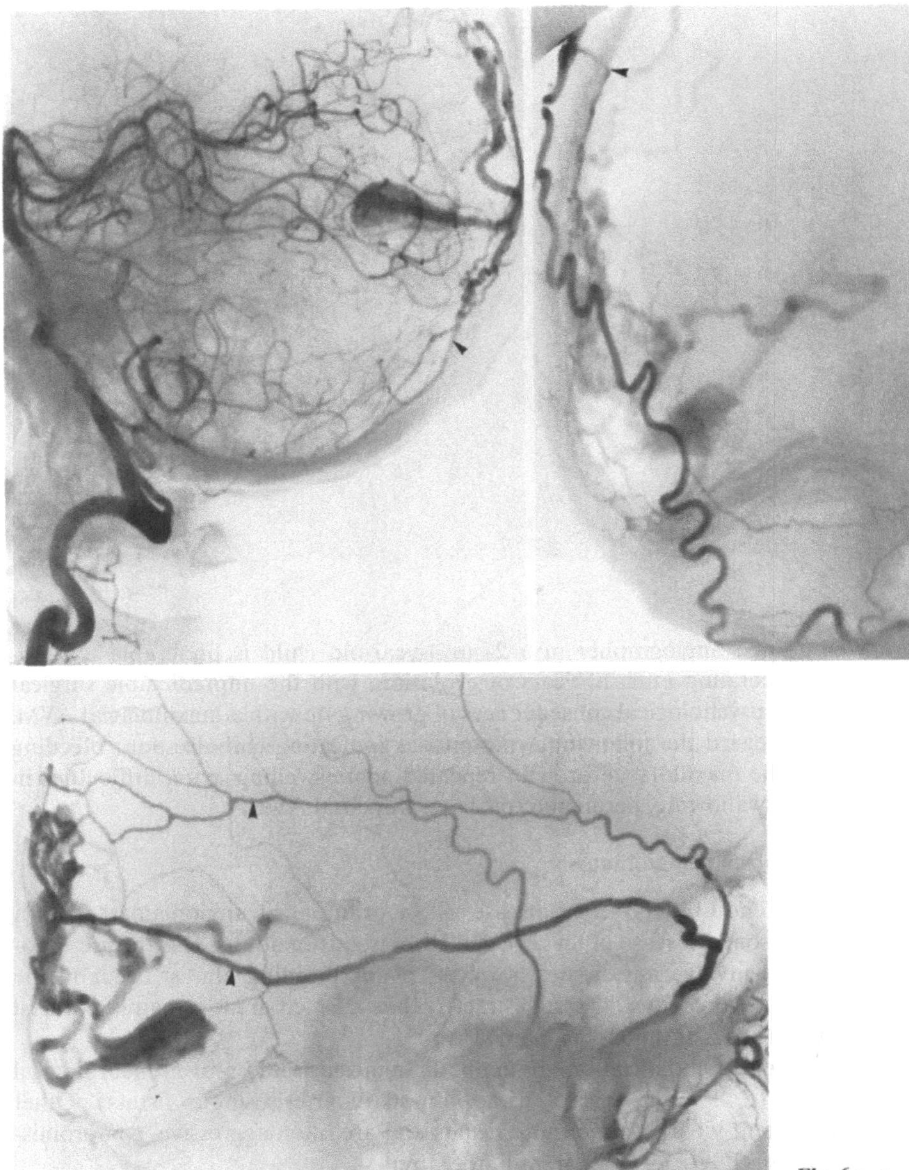

a b c Fig. 6a–c

Fig. 6a–f. Selective study of a dural AVM presenting cerebral symptoms (epilepsy with visual aura). **a** Vertebral injection; **b** right occipital injection; **c** right middle meningeal injection; **d** lateral left occipital view; **e** AP left occipital view; **f** left internal carotid injection. Note the transosseous supply to the malformation (*arrowhead* in **b**, *double arrowheads* in **d, e**). *Single arrowheads* in **a, c–f,** dural feeders of AVM. The middle meningeal constitutes one of the main supply to the AVM, but originates from the left internal carotid artery. Most of the AVM has been embolized with bucrylate but even though the clinical result is good and the nidus has been reached, a faint supply persists from both the vertebral artery and left internal carotid artery

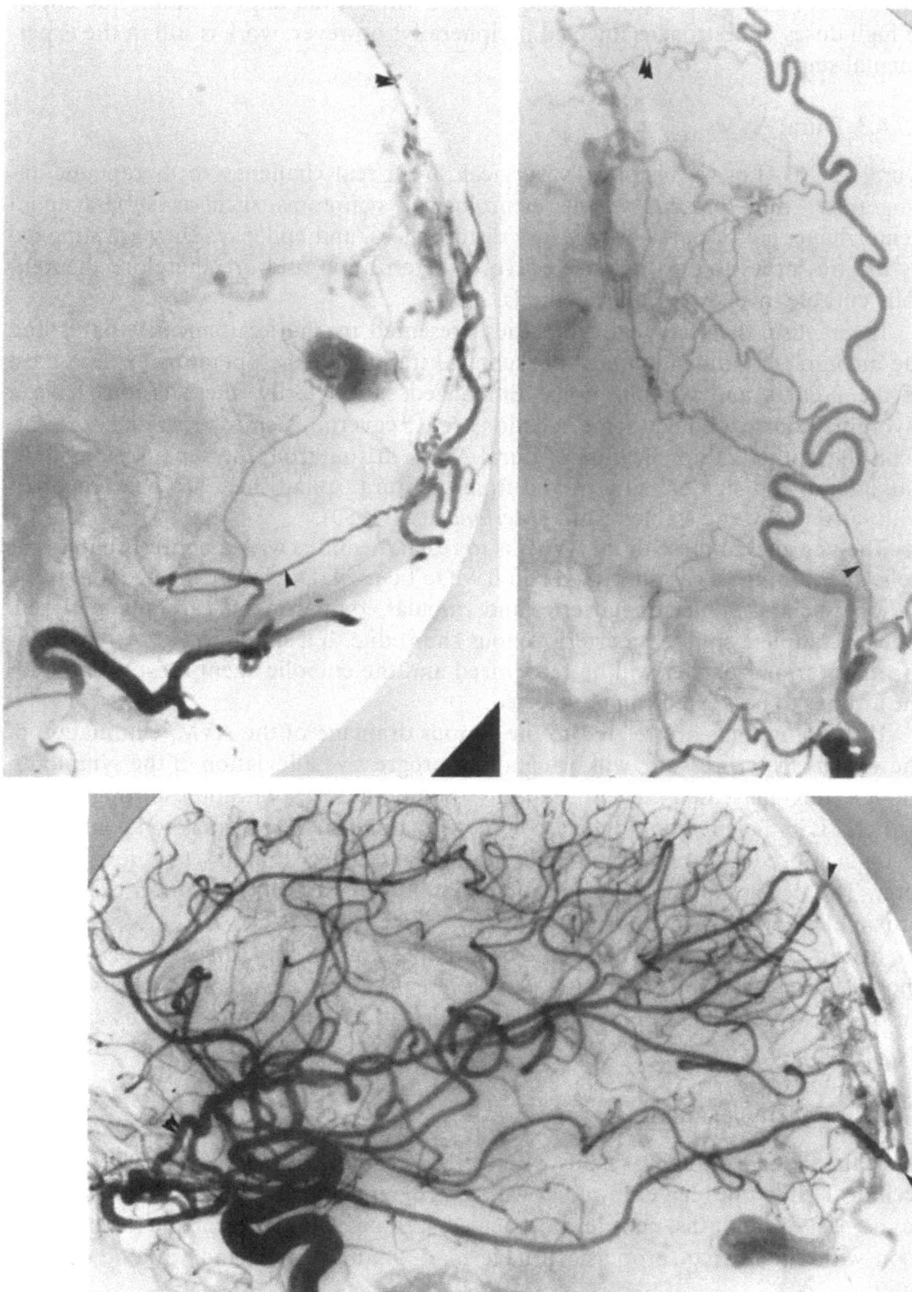

d e f

Fig. 6d–f

should have the same antihemorrhagic effect without the unpredictable side effects of high doses of oestrogens injected peripherally; however, work is still in the experimental stage.

2.7.4.3 Dural AVMs

Dural AVMs (Fig. 6), historically surgical, are a real challenge to therapeutic angiography: they present serious neurological symptoms such as subarachnoid hemorrhage, motor paralysis, sensory disturbances, and epilepsy. They are supplied by arteries accessible to hyperselective catheterization and are therefore theoretically curable by endovascular methods.

In practise, the technical difficulties presented by the anatomical variants and the incomplete radioanatomical or technical training of the operators explain most of the failures and complications. Embolized satisfactorily, these lesions have a favorable course, though some locations (e.g., cavernous sinus) remain more difficult than others. Embolization of dural AVMs arising from the superior longitudinal, lateral, and sigmoid sinuses and from the dural spinal sheet has been reported with satisfactory and stable results (*Merland* et al. 1980).

The key goal in these dural AVMs is to reach the nidus with a nonresorbable embolic agent; in most cases isobutyl will have to be used. Obviously the agent must be radiopaque and the feeding arteries and vascular compartments carefully analyzed. After a complete study, the arteriovenous shunt due to a simple AVM or representing an arteriolar barrier will be recognized and the embolic agent most suitable for the arteries to be treated can be selected.

If the symptoms are related to the venous drainage of the AVM, elimination of the venous hyperpressure, will bring about progressive alleviation of the symptoms, though this may take several months. Sometimes embolization through some pedicles is sufficient to produce a complete anatomical cure thanks to spontaneous secondary occlusion of the others anything from a few minutes to a few months later. The development of collateral circulation shows the failure of an excessively proximal embolization.

In our experience, particles and resorbable emboli give unstable results, and should be reserved for use in slow-flow afferent vessels, as are often observed with an osseous extension in some specific malformations (e.g., sigmoid sinus and temporal bone).

2.7.4.4 Intracranial and Intraspinal AVMs

Since the first encouraging results with Kerber's catheter (*Kerber* et al. 1979), several technical difficulties have slowed down the progress in CNS embolization. However, in the past few months, new developments based on a similar principle (leaking balloon with chamber of propulsion) have made manipulation and embolic delivery safer.

The high degree of technicality involved in the procedure requires great experience and constant practise. Few teams are able to embolize cerebral AVMs "safely" in adults and children. As for the material to be used, it seems that isobutyl in situ is again the best choice for a stable result (*Debrun* et al. 1982; *Epstein* and *Berenstein* 1981).

Some exceptional cases remain embolizable by particles (PVA duramater, Silastic balls) owing to the pumping effect of the AVM; the indications for this method are progressively decreasing.

As with maxillofacial AVMs, the indications for embolization depend largely on the technical skill of the team concerned. Generally, symptomatic lesions with persistent deficits are more often discussed for embolization if they are not operable, but this assessment remains extremely relative. Nonoperable lesions presenting regressive symptoms (deficit, subarachnoid hemorrhage) will be discussed for embolization if they can be reached selectively (Fig. 7).

Peroperative embolization by the direct approach is an additional treatment possibility.

3 Conclusion

This overview of embolization is naturally incomplete and reflects the necessary personal character of the approach. Although valuable experience has been gained, most series are small and clinical follow-up short, and the cases treated 5 years ago cannot be compared to those from 1 year ago, in view of the great improvements achieved. However, with detailed knowledge of anatomy and careful analysis of lesional angioarchitecture, the procedures become safer and the decisions more rational.

It should be kept in mind that there are obviously two ways of studying a lesion angiographically: diagnostically, often with no need for superselective studies, and pretherapeutically, with such studies necessary if an endovascular approach is to be discussed. Global injections and mediocre images will never give enough information to allow the most appropriate choice of therapy and an efficient procedure.

Furthermore, the appearance of a lesion on angiography only interferes with the choice of embolic agent, the indication for treatment and the choice of the approach being at first clinical. Similarly, no lesion has to be treated by embolization only because it is reachable by endovascular procedures or hypervascularized. A clinical goal must be assigned to any type of treatment, including embolization. Thus the absence of the lesion from subsequent angiographic images is no proof of success if not correlated to clinical improvement. In practise, the chances of a given patient receiving embolization therapy depend on where he is treated. Most specialists are underinformed with regard to embolization and some of their assessments are subjective and deprive the patient of the benefit of endovascular treatment. The best

---

Fig. 7a–g see pages 22–25

Fig. 7a–g. A young male presented with acute paraplegia (referred by Prof. Hurth). An initial angiographic exploration (Dr. Gaston) demonstrated a single intraspinal compartment lesion fed by three posterior spinal arteries (**a–c**) and Adamkiewicz' artery (**d**). The treatment in Bicêtre (**e–g**) was carried out by means of selective embolization of one of the posterior spinal feeders with isobutyl (**e**). Note the disappearance of the AVM from the image after injection of the other previously functional feeders (**f–g**). A dramatic improvement was noted: 6 months later the patient was walking, although approximately 20% of the malformation persisted

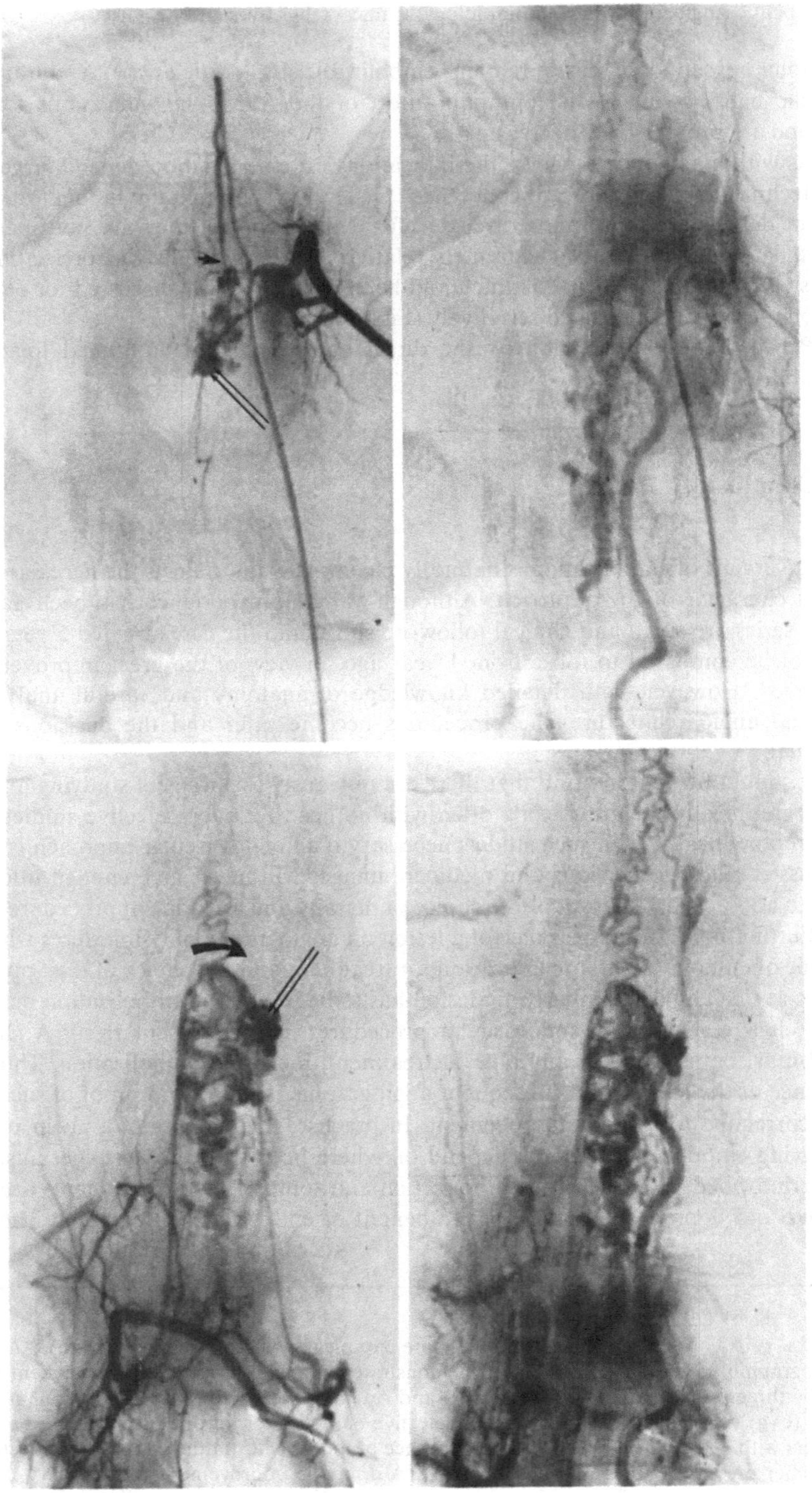

a

b

Fig. 7 a, b. Legend see page 21

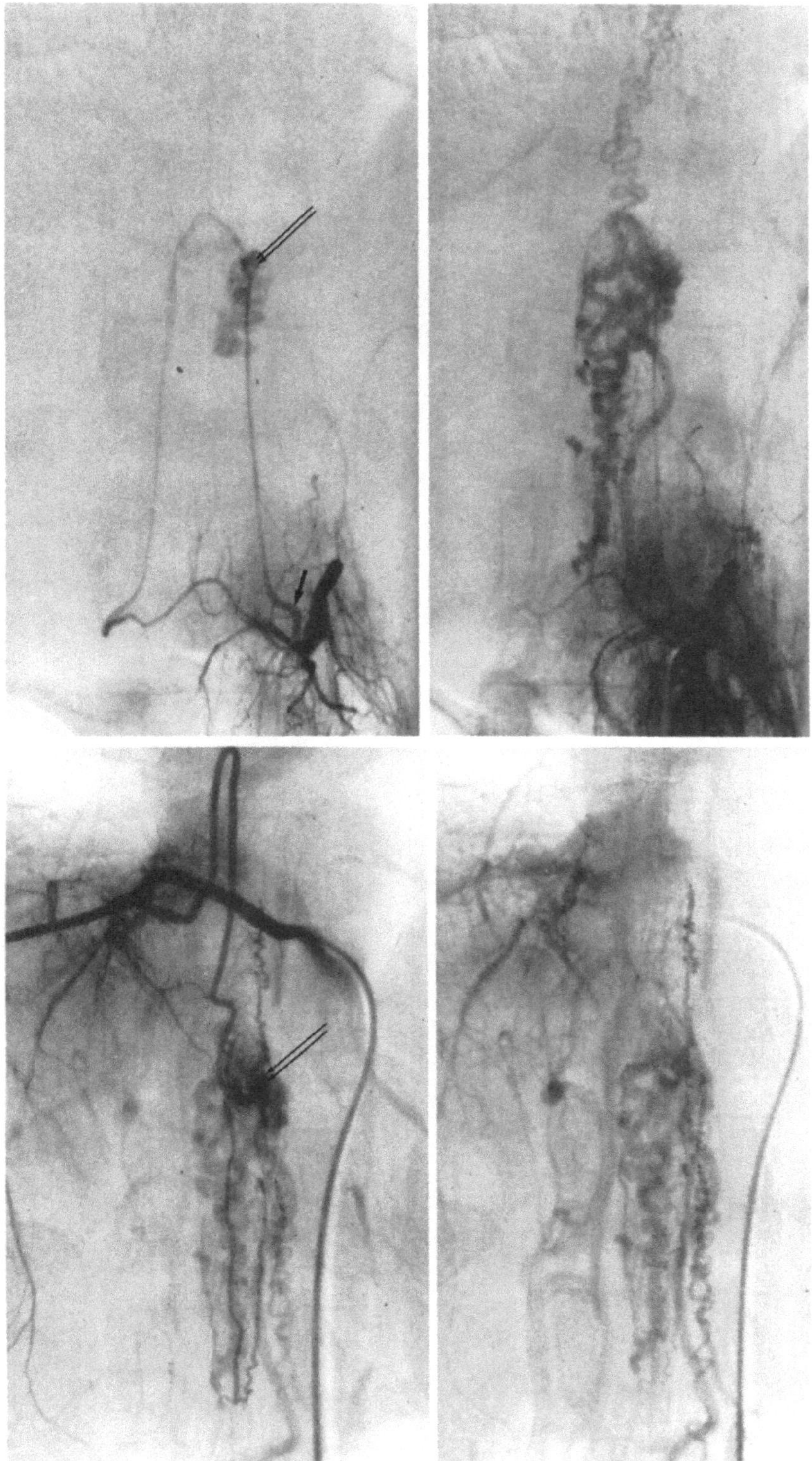

c

d

Fig. 7 c, d. Legend see page 21

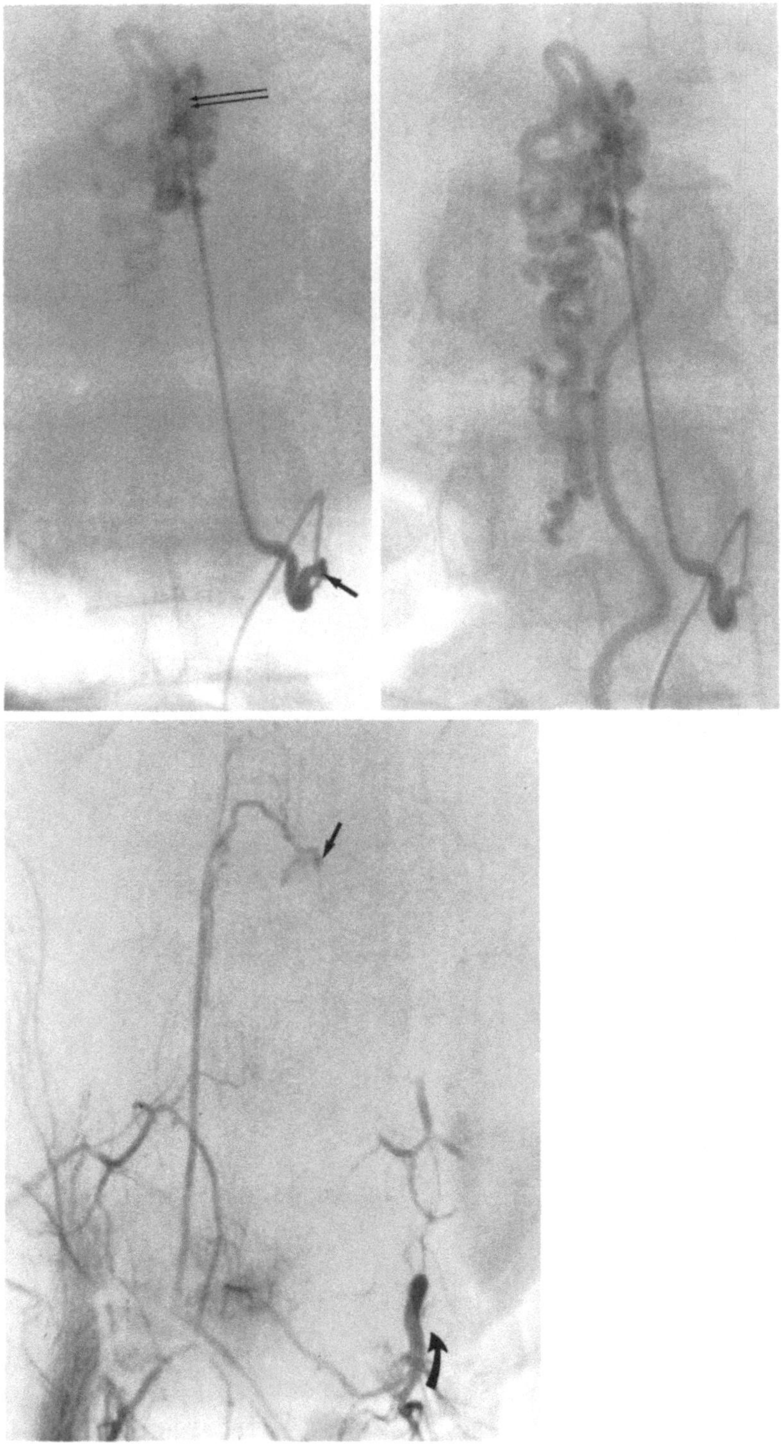

e

f

Fig. 7e, f. Legend see page 21

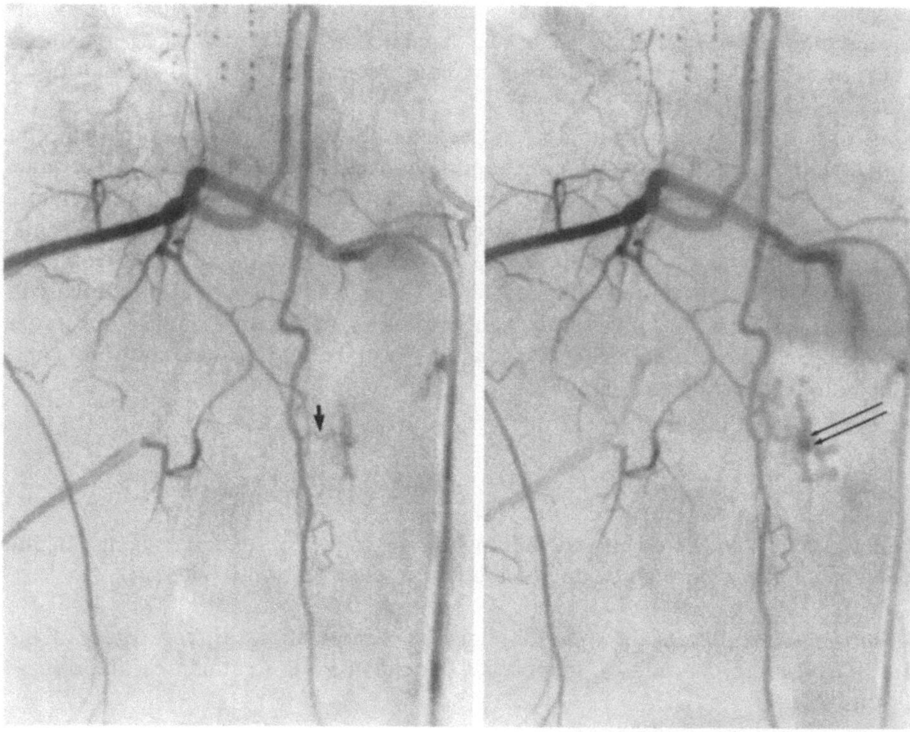

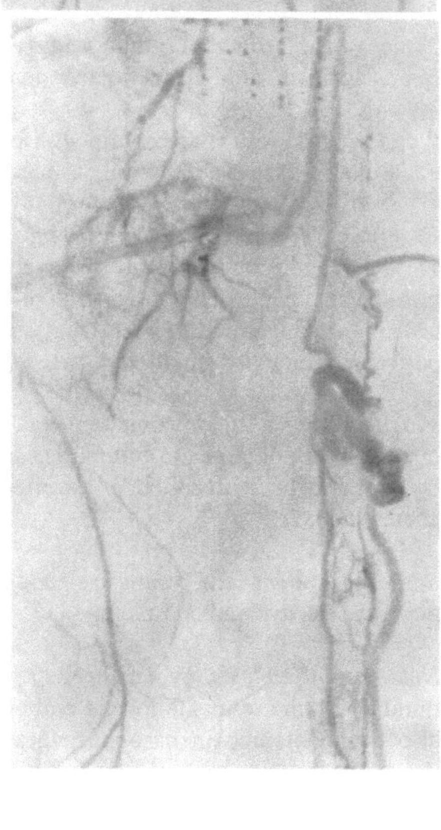

Fig. 7g. Legend see page 21

example is probably given by traumatic caroticocavernous fistula, which are too often operated upon, overlooking the fact that in more than 50% of cases, embolization by means of a detachable balloon can preserve the internal carotid artery (*Debrun* et al. 1981 a).

It is plain that both neurologists and neurosurgeons can examine a patient, but no one would accept having a brain tumor removed by a neurologist. In the same way, both diagnostic and therapeutic neuroradiologists can read carotid or vertebral angiograms, but embolization is obviously done preferably by full-time therapeutic specialists. There is as much difference between diagnostic and therapeutic angiographic discussions as between medical and surgical discussions. This emphasizes the need for specific training within neuroradiology to permit embolization to develop, take its place among neurospecialities, and be carried out safely by competent and responsible angiographers.

4 Summary

Embolization is today crucial to therapeutic angiography, and knowledge of the beneficial effects which can be obtained helps in selection of suitable cases.

Hemorrhage. Hemostatsis can be obtained in almost all cases, regardless of the cause of bleeding. Stability of hemostasis depends on the treatment of the disease responsible.

Tumor Mass. Reduction in tumor mass can be helpful in mechanical compression. It can be achieved in highly cellular lesions; hypervascularity is not a precondition.

Pain. The best results are obtained in pain related to tumor mass. Some relief of intractable headaches and neuralgias has been observed.

Evolution, Malignancy, and Recurrence. These depend on the quantity of tumor tissue destroyed. Obviously any recurrence corresponding to incomplete surgical removal will benefit from preoperative embolization. Good results are obtained in lesions evolving with the menstrual cycle. Palliative treatment of tumors has been performed, though without adequate follow-up.

Vascular Bruits. The outcome depends on the cause of the bruits. The most rewarding results are obtained in traumatic carotico-cavernous fistulas, which should never be operated on first. Good or excellent results are observed in dural AVMs and aneurysms.

Secreting Lesions. The results are good if the infusion or embolization has been sufficiently selective and complete.

Neurological Deficits. When the deficits are related to venous hyperpressure in a dural AVM, the results following embolization are especially rewarding. Success has also been obtained in nasopharyngeal angiofibromas. Paragangliomas, otorhinolaryngological cancers, maxillofacial, intracerebral, and intraspinal AVMs, and Rendu-Osler-Weber disease.

Embolization can form a treatment in itself or a part of the overall treatment plan. In either case, the responsibility for the decision on therapy lies with the angiographer, who must not transfer it to the referring clinician. The decision requires clinical, anatomical, and technical knowledge, with methodical analysis of the clinical information. Angiographic images should not be treated, but areas of abnormal function: Disappearance of a lesion from the image is neither goal nor guarantee of success. Clinical improvement should be behind every indication for embolization.

References

Berenstein A (1980) Flow controlled silicone fluid embolization. AJNR 1:161–166

Berenstein A, Kricheff, II (1979a) Catheter and material for transarterial embolization. I. Catheters. Radiology 132:619–630

Berenstein A, Kricheff II (1979b) Catheter and material for transarterial embolization. II. Materials.Radiology 132:631–639

Berenstein A, Kricheff II (1981) Microembolization techniques of vascular occlusion: radiologic, pathologic and clinical correlation. AJNR 2:261–267

Berenstein A, Kricheff II, Ransohoff J (1980) Carotid cavernous fistulas: intraarterial treatment. AJNR 1:449–457

Brem S (1976) The role of vascular proliferation in the growth of brain tumors. Clinical neurosurgery. Williams & Wilkins, Baltimore

Debrun G, Lacour P, Caron JP et al. (1978) Detachable balloon and calibrated leak balloon technique in the treatment of cerebral vascular lesions. J Neurosurg 49:635–649

Debrun G, Lacour P, Vinuela F, Fox A, Drake C, Caron J (1981a) Treatment of 54 traumatic carotid-cavernous fistulas. J Neurosurg 55:678–692

Debrun G, Fox A, Peerless S et al. (1981b) Giant unclippable aneurysm: treatment with detachable balloons. AJNR 2:267–273

Debrun G, Vinuela F, Fox A, Drake C (1982) Embolization of cerebral arteriovenous malformations with bucrylate: experience in 46 cases. J Neurosurg 56:615–627

Djindjian R, Merland JJ (1978) Superselective arteriography of the external carotid artery, vol 1. Springer, Berlin Heidelberg New York

Doyon D, Lasjaunias P, Manelfe C et al. (1978) Analysis of the complications of therapeutic angiography: review of 800 embolizations in the cranio-cephalic area. IXème Symposium Neuroradiologicum, Wiesbaden

Epstein F, Berenstein A (1981) Pediatric vascular anomalies: combined neurosurgical and neuroradiologic intervention. In: American Society for Pediatric Neurosurgery (ed) Pediatric neurosurgery I. Karger, Basel, pp 49–68

Fellus P, Lasjaunias P, Deffez JP (1979) Le contact bilabial: but à atteindre dans les traitements des rétromandibulies. Actual Odontostomatol 128:733–746

Kerber CW, Bank WO, Cromwell LD (1979) Calibrated leak balloon microcatheter: a device for arterial exploration and occlusive therapy. AJR 132:207–212

Kunstlinger F, Brunelle F, Chaumont P, Doyon D (1981) Review vascular occlusive agents. AJR 136:151–156

Lasjaunias P (1981) Cranio-facial and upper cervical arteries, vol I. Anatomy, normal angiographic aspects. Williams & Wilkins, Baltimore

Lasjaunias P (1983) Cranio-facial and upper cervical arteries, vol II. Collateral circulation and angiographic protocols. Williams & Wilkins, Baltimore

Lasjaunias P, Doyon D (1980) Les malformations de la cavité buccale. J Neuroradiol 4:243–270

Lasjaunias P, Doyon D (1981) Angiographie diagnostique et thérapeutique en neuropédiatrie. Ann Otol Rhinol Laryngol 98:625–628

Lasjaunias P, Picard L, Manelfe C et al. (1980) Angiofibrome nasopharyngien. Revue de 53 cas avec embolisation. Place de l'angiographie pré-thérapeutique: hypothèses physio-pathogéniques. J Neuroradiol 7:73–95
Lasjaunias P, Menu Y, Bonnel D, Doyon D (1981) Les paragangliomes non chromaffines de la tête et du cou. J Neuroradiol 8:281–299
Luessenhop AJ, Presber JH (1975) Surgical embolization of cerebral arteriovenous malformations through internal carotid and vertebral arteries. Long term results. J Neurosurg 42:443–451
Madoule PH, Trampont PH, Doyon D et al. (1981) Expérimentation chez le chien de microbilles utilisables en angiographie thérapeutique. J Radiol 62:457–462
Manelfe C, Picard L, Bonafe A et al. (1978) Embolisations et occlusions par ballonnets dans les processus tumoraux: sept années d'expérience. Neuroradiology 16:395–398
Merland JJ, Riche MA, Chiras J (1980) Fistules arterio-veineuses intracanalaires, extra-médullaires à drainage veineux médullaire. J Neuroradiol 7:271–320
Merland JJ, Melki JP, Chiras J et al. (1981) L'embolisation d'hémostase: possibilités et perspectives: 190 observations. Nouv Presse Med 10:1385–1387
Moret J, Lasjaunias P, Theron J (1980) Vascular compartments and territories of tympano-jugular glomic tumors. J Belge Radiol 63:321–337
Picard L, Lepoire J, Montaut J et al. (1974a) Endarterial occlusion of carotid cavernous sinus fistulas using a balloon-tipped catheter. Neuroradiology 8:5–10
Picard L, Andre JM, Djindjian R et al. (1974b) Angiographie superselective et embolisation des localisations oto-rhinolaryngologiques de l'angiomatose de Rendu-Osler. J Neuroradiol 4:251–356
Picard L, Manelfe C, Roland J, Treil J, Andre JM, De Ker Saint Gilly A, Morel C (1978) Embolisations et occlusions par ballonnets dans les lésions vasculaires crânio-faciales. Neuroradiology 16:393–394
Riche MC, Chiras J, Melki JP, Merland JJ (1979) Place de l'embolisation dans les épistaxis graves. J Neuroradiol 6:207–220
Serbinenko FA (1974) Balloon catheterization and occlusion of major cerebral vessels. J Neurosurg 41:125–145
Serbinenko FA (1978) Six hundred endovascular neurosurgical procedures in vascular pathology. A ten year experience. Acta Neurochir [Suppl] 28:310–311
Tazi Z, Lasjaunias P, Doyon D (1981) Malformations vasculaires de la face et du scalp. Ann Otol Rhinol Laryngol 98:625–628
Vinters HV, Debrun G, Kaufmann JCE et al. (1981) Pathology of arteriovenous malformations embolized with isobutyl-2-cyanoacrylate (bucrylate). Report of 2 cases. J Neurosurg 55:819–825

Densitometric Investigations of Renal Perfusion by Dynamic X-Ray Computed Tomography*

U. Reiser, J. Buck, and F. Heuck[1]

1 Introduction

X-ray computed tomography (CT) not only has the potential to provide information on the topography, form, size, contour, and structure of the kidney without surgical intervention, but also, by means of sequential CT studies, allows conclusions to be drawn on the normal and pathologic perfusion of this excretory organ. Sequential CT can be defined as a series of CT scans taken in the same body slice so that changes in enhancement after intravenous contrast medium injection can be evaluated qualitatively as well as quantitatively. Unlike in other parenchymal organs, sequential CT of the kidneys has the advantage that the symmetry of the urinary system admits comparison between the affected and the normal side. Furthermore, the segmentary construction of the kidney allows localization of a disorder.

The high spatial resolution and the improved sensitivity of X-ray CT at low contrasts enable analysis of the kinetics of intravenously injected contrast medium boluses in the kidney by means of fast image sequences.

A large number of authors have applied sequential CT to investigation and description of the enhancement of the kidneys after administration of contrast medium. A general theoretical analysis of contrast medium kinetics was published by *Axel* (1980). Other authors have mostly investigated the practical aspects of the ki-

* This research was supported by the Deutsche Forschungsgemeinschaft (German Research Organisation)

1 Radiologisches Institut des Katharinenhospitals der Stadt Stuttgart, Kriegsbergstraße 60, D-7000 Stuttgart 1. Submitted for publication in April 1983

netics of contrast medium. *Brennan* et al. (1979 a, b) investigated the enhancement in the renal cortex and medulla of dogs. They administered different concentrations and amounts of contrast media manually at a flow of about 2 ml/s and obtained different levels of enhancement. *Ono* et al. (1980) also used dogs to register the enhancement in the plasma after various modes of contrast medium administration – drip infusion and bolus injection (1 ml/s). *Gardeur* et al. (1980) studied the pharmacokinetics of contrast media in dogs and man after bolus injection at a flow of about 1.5 ml/s, and *Ishikawa* et al. (1981) analyzed dynamic CT curves of the kidneys after injection of contrast medium at a flow of 2.7 ml/s. *Baert* et al. (1980) examined the contrast enhancement by bolus technique but did not define the injection flow used. Other authors injected between 50 ml (*Heinz* et al. 1980) and 100 ml (*Hübener* and *Klott* 1980) of contrast medium, either by hand or mechanical injector (*Heinz* et al. 1980), with injection flows between 4 and 15 ml/s (*Heller* et al. 1981 a, b).

As this small list shows, there is wide variation in what different authors understand as a suitable bolus injection of contrast materials for dynamic CT investigations of the kidneys, and this makes it difficult to compare the results and enhancement curves demonstrated. It therefore had been our aim to determine how the mode of injection (flow rate, volume, and concentration of contrast medium) influences the resulting enhancement. With the aid of systematic investigations, a recommendation for a standard injection mode was worked out. It thus became possible to compare enhancement curves obtained after standard bolus injection not only qualitatively, but also quantitatively, and to correlate the parameters obtained with clinical findings.

2 Material and Methods

The investigations described in this report were carried out on a total of 51 subjects, including both individuals without pathologic findings and patients suffering from renovascular hypertension where contrast medium injection was indicated clinically. The studies were performed using a Siemens Somatom SF scanner (Siemens AG, Erlangen, West Germany). With this type of whole body scanner it is possible to produce sequential tomograms every 10 s with a scanning time of 4.8 s. The level of the transverse slice through the kidneys should be chosen with the help of an AP digital radiograph – a Topogram. To enable a comparison of the left and right kidneys, the tomograms should include both renal pelvises (Fig. 1) All tomograms of a sequence must be exposed during expiration, so that the same slice of the kidneys will always be scanned (Fig. 2) despite the respiratory movement of the abdominal organs.

The temporal resolution, six images per minute, is not very high, but is sufficient for enhancement studies of the kidneys, where no rapid changes in density occur after intravenous injection of contrast medium. The sampling speed can be augmented with the aid of a segmental or image-split reconstruction. In this mode, images of different temporal centers of gravity are reconstructed by using overlapping segments of a single 360° scan.

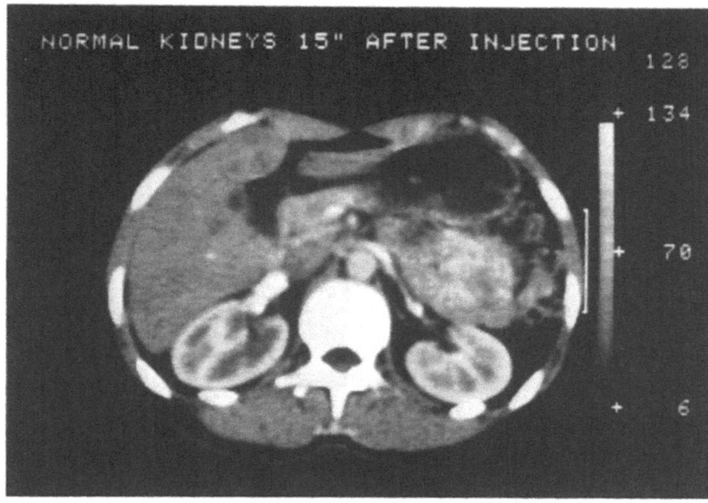

Fig. 1. CT scan at the level of the kidneys 15 s after intravenous bolus injection of contrast medium

The improved spatial resolution of third-generation X-ray CT enables the densities of the renal cortex, medulla, and papillae to be evaluated separately. The densitometric evaluation of the tomographic sequences was carried out with the aid of the scanner-independent image-processing system Evaluscop (Siemens AG), which allows the description of regions of interest (ROIs) within the reconstructed images for quantitative evaluation.

The magnification of the images facilitates the separate analysis of the cortex and medulla (Fig. 3). Distinguishing between perfusion in the cortex and in the medulla is of importance, as pathologic insufficiencies of the kidney can affect these areas independently. The number of picture elements (pixels) included in an ROI after magnification, e.g., 300 pixels for the renal cortex, is sufficient for evaluation of the mean density and the separation of minor differences in the tissue density. Each ROI is defined manually for each tomogram of a series. This procedure is troublesome and time consuming, but avoids the faults in measurement and false conclusions which would arise if the same ROI were superimposed on all images, as small variations in the respiratory movement of the kidneys cannot be totally avoided even if the tomograms are exposed only during expiration.

As precise discrimination of the renal medulla from the renal papillae can be difficult, only the maximum density values in the medulla are used to compute the time-density curves for this area.

In the renal pelvis too, only the maximum values are used for quantitative evaluation, as the mixture of the residual urine in the pelvis and the contrast urine excreted into it can be inhomogeneous (Fig. 2).

After evaluation of the density values within corresponding areas in all images of a series, time-density curves can be computed. In order to obtain the enhancement due to the injected contrast medium, the curves have to be normalized to values measured before application of contrast medium. This enables quantitative com-

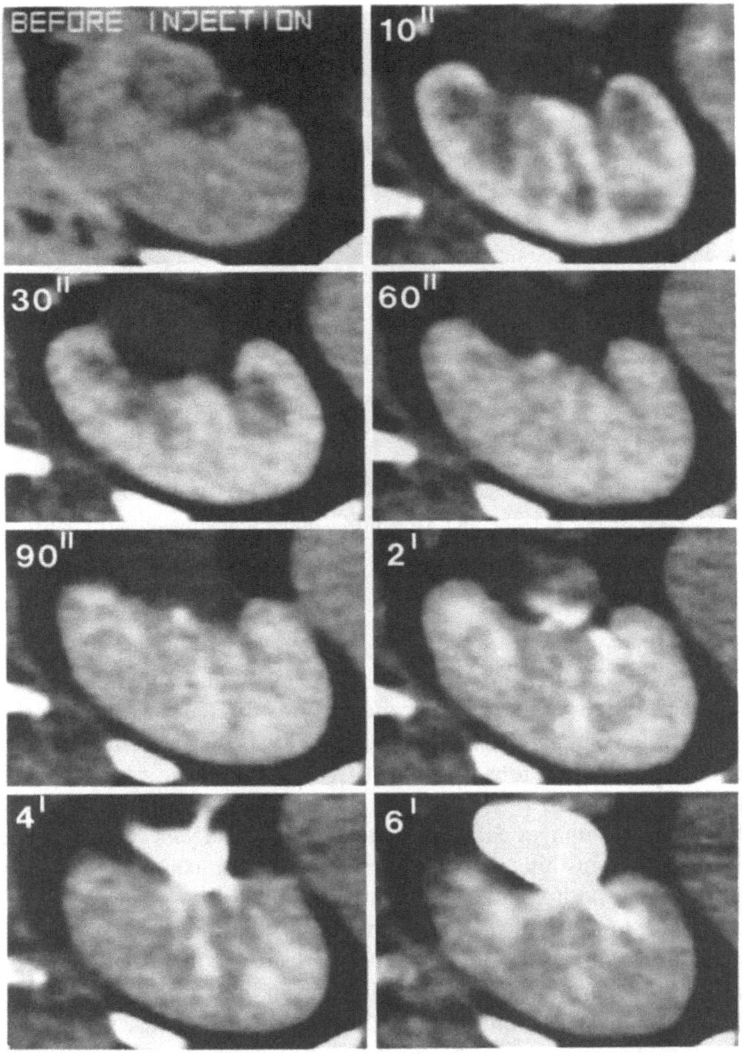

Fig. 2. Tomogram sequence of a normal left kidney after intravenous bolus injection. The renal cortex is opacified 10 s after the end of the injection, and by 90 s a homogeneous density distribution is attained. After 2 min, excretion of contrast urine into the renal pelvis commences. After 4 min, mixing of contrast urine and residual urine in the pelvis can be observed

parison of the enhancement curves of corresponding parts of the kidneys. The enhancement can be expressed in Hounsfield units (HU) or in ΔHU, the difference between the densities before and after the administration of contrast medium. As can be proved in a model experiment using a series of plastic rods filled with different concentrations of contrast medium (Telebrix 300, Byk Gulden), the relationship between the attenuation (expressed in HU) and the contrast medium concentration (expressed in milligrams iodine per milliliter) is linear in the range of enhancement occurring in the kidneys (Fig. 4). The factor to convert HU to milligrams

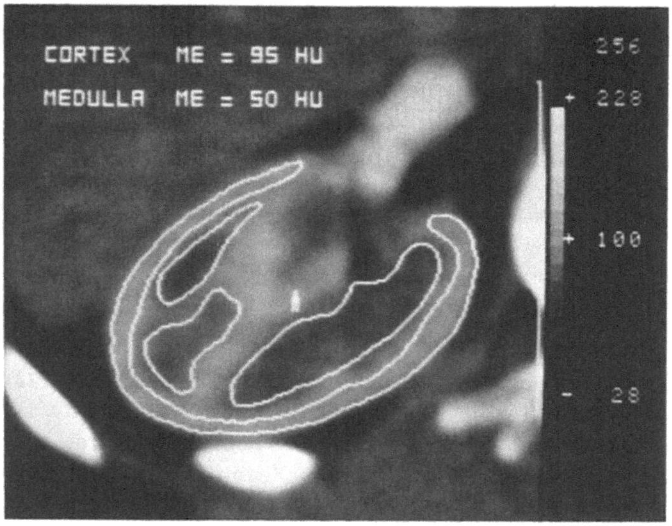

Fig. 3. Magnified CT image of the right kidney. ROIs of the cortex and medulla are superimposed for enhancement measurement. ME, mean density

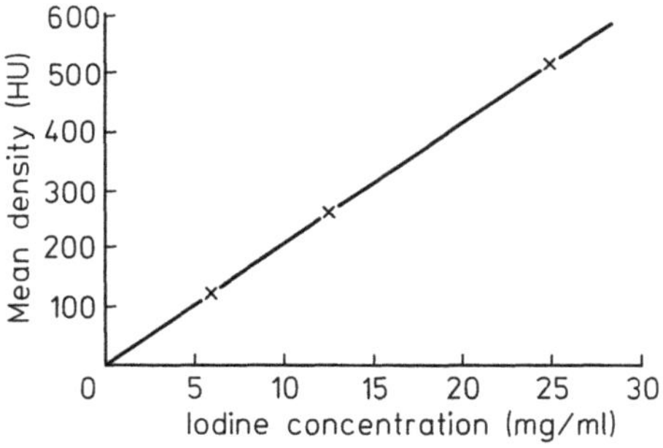

Fig. 4. The linear relationship between contrast medium concentration and the corresponding attenuation. The enhancement measured in an ROI can be converted into the absolute contrast medium concentration using the equation $c = 0.049 \cdot \Delta HU$

iodine per milliliter was found to be 0.049. Thus an increase in enhancement of 1 HU corresponds to an augmentation of 49 μg iodine/ml blood and the enhancement expressed as ΔHU can be converted into the absolute contrast medium concentration c expressed in milligrams iodine per milliliter using the relation $c = 0.049 \cdot \Delta HU$.

3 Influence of the Mode of Injection on Bolus Geometry

When iodine-containing contrast medium is injected into the cubital vein, injection parameters like contrast medium volume, flow rate and concentration influence the geometry of the contrast medium bolus. The excretion potential of the kidneys is independent of mode of injection, but basic changes in bolus geometry caused by the mode of injection can make efficient measurement and a quantitative evaluation of

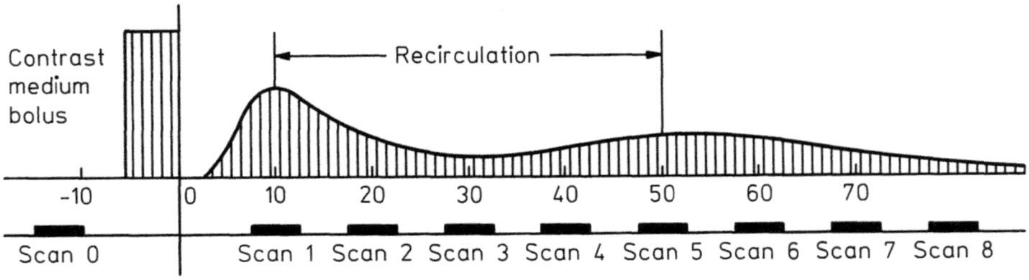

Fig. 5. Temporal succession of intravenous injection of contrast medium and scans for a sequential CT study demonstrating the general enhancement in the abdominal aorta

the resulting enhancement more difficult and can prevent the comparison of results from different patients. It is therefore necessary to study the influence of the mode of injection on bolus geometry and to define a standard.

Bolus geometry after injection of contrast medium into the cubital vein can best be studied in the upper abdominal aorta. The enhancement in the aorta is of particular interest for quantitative evaluations because the time-density curve measured here can be understood mathematically as the input function to all distal parts of the body, for example the excretory system. The enhancement curves registered in the aorta then represent the response function of the system to the input bolus.

For study of the influence of mode of injection on bolus geometry, 18 patients with normal cardiovascular values – most of them receiving radiotherapy – were selected if the normal CT-study indicated the necessity for contrast medium injection. The injections were performed using a hydraulic high-pressure injector controlled by a digital processor, developed at the Institute of Biomedical Engineering of the University of Stuttgart for special angiographic examinations. After a reference tomogram prior to the injection of contrast medium, the sequential tomograms were performed every 10 s with a scanning time of 4.8 s during the 1st min after injection. Thereafter the same slice was scanned every 30 s until the end of the examination 6 min after injection. Figure 5 shows the temporal succession of injection and scans, with the general enhancement in the abdominal aorta.

In studying the influence of mode of injection on bolus geometry, the effects of variations in contrast medium flow rate, volume, and concentration were observed.

Flow Rate. Volume (30 ml) and concentration (300 mg iodine/ml) of contrast medium (Telebrix 300) were kept constant. Flow rate varied between 4 and 10 ml con-

→

Fig. 6. Time-density graph showing the influence of injection flow on the enhancement (averaged values) in the abdominal aorta. The injected contrast medium volume (30 ml) and concentration (300 mg iodine/ml) were kept constant. –·–·– , 4 ml/s; ——, 6 ml/s; – – –, 8 ml/s; . . ., 10 ml/s

Fig. 7. Time-density graph showing the influence of contrast medium volume injected on enhancement in the abdominal aorta. Injection flow (6 ml/s) and contrast medium concentration (300 mg iodine/ml) were kept constant. ——, 30 ml; –·–·– , 40 ml; – – – –, 60 ml

Fig. 8. Time-density graph showing the influence of the contrast medium concentration on enhancement. Injection flow (6 ml/s) and injected volume (30 ml) were kept constant. —— 300 mg iodine/ml; –·–·– 380 mg iodine/ml

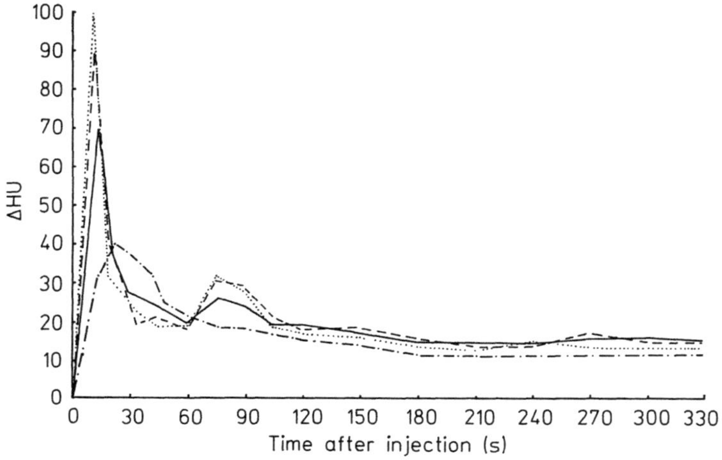

Fig. 6

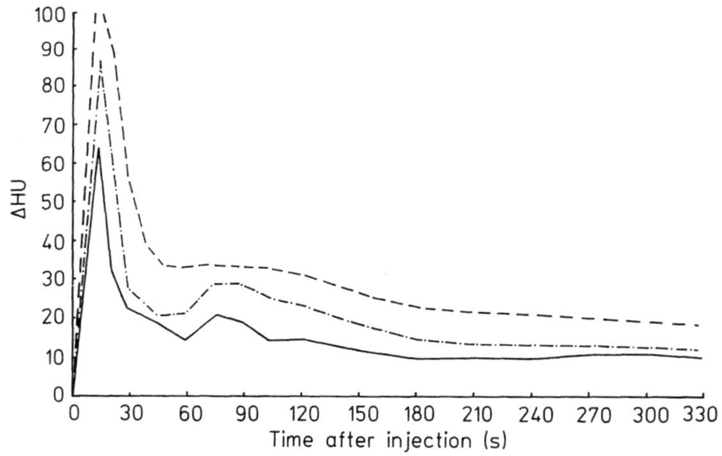

Fig. 7

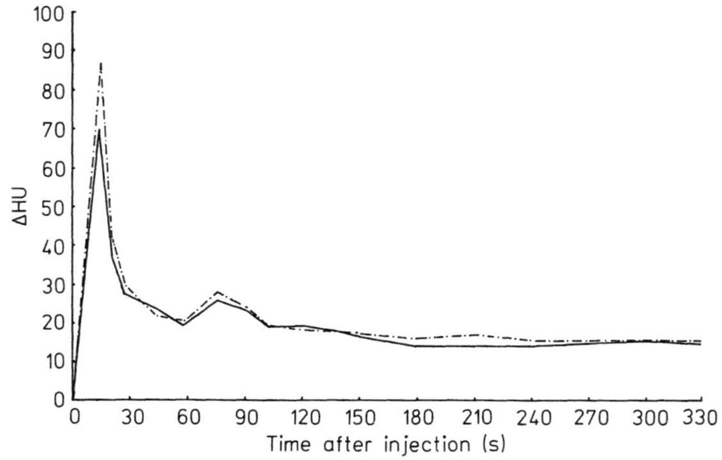

Fig. 8

trast medium/s. It could be observed that augmentation of the flow rate leads to a "sharp" contrast medium bolus – the gradient of the density increases and the enhancement reaches its maximum more rapidly (Fig. 6). In model experiments performed with a special circulation simulator (*Decker* et al. 1983), doubling of flow rate caused a linear increase of enhancement up to a rate of 30 ml/s. In contrast, in vivo studies showed that augmentation of the rate to more than 8 ml/s does not increase enhancement to the same degree.

Volume. Concentration (300 mg iodine/ml) and flow rate (6 ml/s) were kept constant. Volumes of 30, 40, and 60 ml were injected, with corresponding injection times. Augmentation of the injected volume results in higher maximum density values. The gradient of the enhancement increases, but the initial maximum concentration is reached later (Fig. 7). The decrease of enhancement is exponential, but less rapid if a high amount of contrast medium is injected.

Concentration. Contrast medium volume (30 ml) and flow rate (6 ml/s) were kept constant. Concentration was varied from 300 mg iodine/ml (Telebrix 300) to 380 mg iodine/ml (Telebrix 380). A significant correlation between concentration and enhancement could be observed (Fig. 8). The increase in the measured iodine concentration in the abdominal aorta after injection into the cubital vein is approximately 10%. The injection of highly concentrated contrast medium does not affect the arrival time of the initial density peak, but the gradient of the curve increases.

These analyses demonstrate that the geometry of a contrast medium bolus injected into the cubital vein and measured in the abdominal aorta is affected not only by individual circulation parameters, but also by contrast medium flow rate, volume, and concentration. The enhancement and the maximum density of a contrast medium bolus passing the aorta are influenced by both flow rate and concentration of the contrast medium. These findings correlate well with the tendencial results obtained by *Brennan* et al. (1979 a, b) and *Ono* et al. (1980) in animal studies when they varied the volume and concentration of contrast medium injected.

As our studies show, the width of a bolus is determined predominantly by the volume; it is obvious that a higher volume increases the total injection time when injected at the same flow rate as a lower volume.

The most significant finding of our studies is that a flow rate of more than 8 ml/s does not lead to a significantly greater degree of enhancement in the aorta. It has to be assumed that in this case the lungs work as a buffer. Thus it is not of any great advantage to introduce contrast medium into the cubital vein at a rate of more than 8 ml/s; this only causes unnecessary side effects.

The study shows that if a sharp bolus is required, injection of 32 ml of highly concentrated contrast medium (300 mg iodine/ml or more) at a rate of 8 ml/s gives the best enhancement, sufficient in most cases for computer-aided quantitative evaluations. In our hospital we reduced the rate to 6 ml/s with a volume of 30 ml; a slow rate does not harm patients with weak veins, and a low volume has no ill effects on those suffering from reduced renal function.

4 Quantitative Studies of Renal Perfusion

CT angiography and dynamic or sequential CT have not only been applied to studying the enhancement after contrast medium injection in healthy kidneys or parts of them, e.g., the renal cortex (*Ishikawa* et al. 1981; *Hübener* 1978). *Heinz* et al. (1980) recorded enhancement curves of dog infarct kidneys, and *Walz* et al. (1982) studied the enhancement of the cortex, medulla, and renal pelvis before and after reflux and/or obstruction in minipigs, but did not relate their findings to findings in humans.

The precondition for assessment of pathologic changes in kidney perfusion and the associated excretion of contrast materials is a knowledge of these activities in normally functioning kidneys. After a standard injection of contrast medium into the cubital vein (30 ml at 6 ml/s; 300 mg iodine/ml), enhancement curves have been evaluated for the different kidney areas: cortex, medulla, papillae, and pelvis, as described in Sect. 2.

Time-density curves have also been evaluated for the abdominal aorta and the vena cava at the level of the kidneys. We agree with other authors (*Ishikawa* et al. 1981; *Burgener* and *Hamlin* 1981; *Heinz* et al. 1980; *Hübener* and *Klott* 1980) that the measurement of enhancement in the aorta as the input function for the excretory system is indispensable for interpretation of curves showing renal function. The enhancements in the liver and spleen do not appear to give extra information about the excretory potential of the kidneys.

4.1 Normal Findings

The enhancement in the kidneys of patients with normal circulation parameters and normal renal function, computed as time-density curves from CT sequences, is plotted in Fig. 9.

Abdominal Aorta. The contrast enhancement in the aorta at the level of the kidneys exhibits a fast, high initial peak about 10 s after the end of injection of contrast medium into the cubital vein. The mean maximum iodine concentration evaluated for 18 patients was 3.5 mg iodine/ml blood, corresponding to an enhancement of 70 HU. Because of the recirculation of the opacified blood through the major circulation system, a second rise in density can be observed, reaching on average 40% of the concentration of the initial peak and followed by further recirculation waves of decreasing amplitude.

Renal Cortex. A rapid increase in density occurs, reaching its maximum 10–15 s after the end of the injection. This peak results from the initial influx of opacified blood into the cortex and is related to the initial enhancement peak in the aorta. The subsequent decrease, similar to that in the aorta, is superimposed on the commencement of the filtration of iodine. The gradient of the decrease is therefore not as great as in the aorta, and after about 50 s the filtration effect predominates, resulting in another increase in density whose maximum is reached after 2 min. Thereafter the enhancement decreases slowly as the injected iodine is excreted.

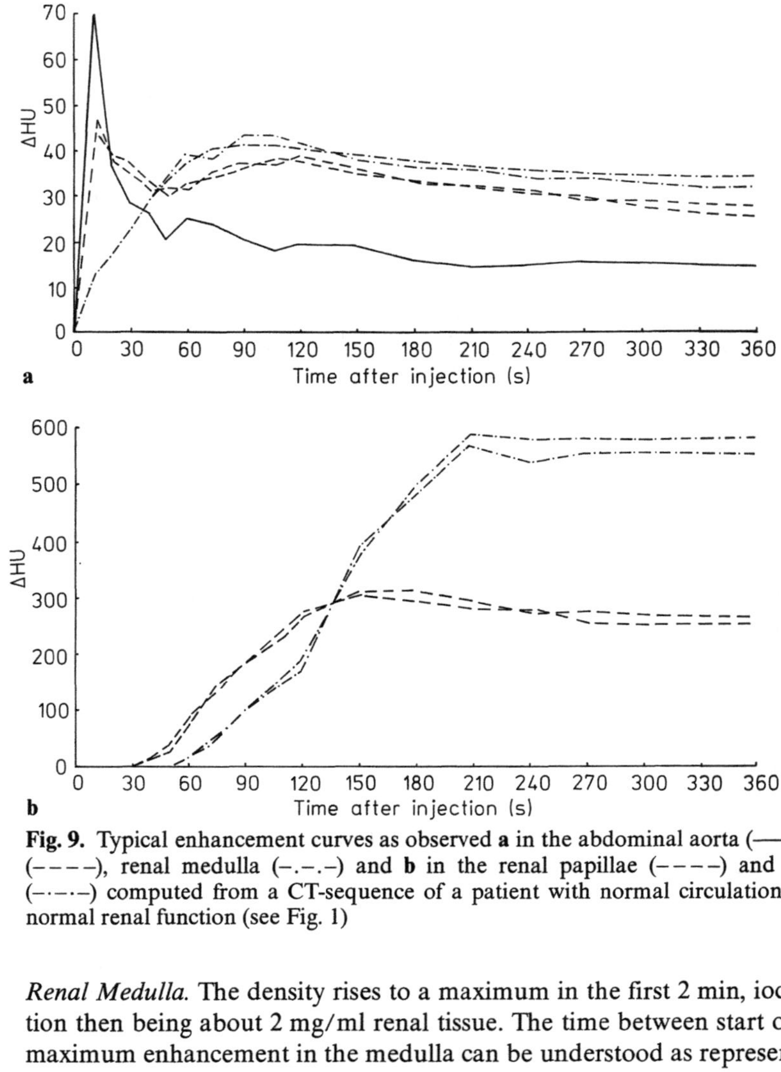

Fig. 9. Typical enhancement curves as observed **a** in the abdominal aorta (———), renal cortex (– – – –), renal medulla (–.–.–) and **b** in the renal papillae (– – – –) and the renal pelvis (–·–·–) computed from a CT-sequence of a patient with normal circulation parameters and normal renal function (see Fig. 1)

Renal Medulla. The density rises to a maximum in the first 2 min, iodine concentration then being about 2 mg/ml renal tissue. The time between start of injection and maximum enhancement in the medulla can be understood as representing the blood filtration capability of the kidney. The decrease after maximum enhancement also reflects this potential; 6 min after injection, enhancement is reduced to an average of 30 HU, corresponding to an iodine concentration of 1.5 mg/ml renal tissue, about 75% of the maximum density value.

Renal Papillae. The increase in enhancement begins about 40 s after injection. After about 150 s the maximum density of 300 HU is reached, corresponding to an iodine concentration of 15 mg/ml.

Renal Pelvis. The influx of contrast urine can be observed after 1 min. The density of the filtrated urine increases within 3 min after injection to 600 HU, corresponding to 30 mg iodine/ml urine, or to even higher values – the iodine concentration can go above the maximum measurable density of + 1000 HU.

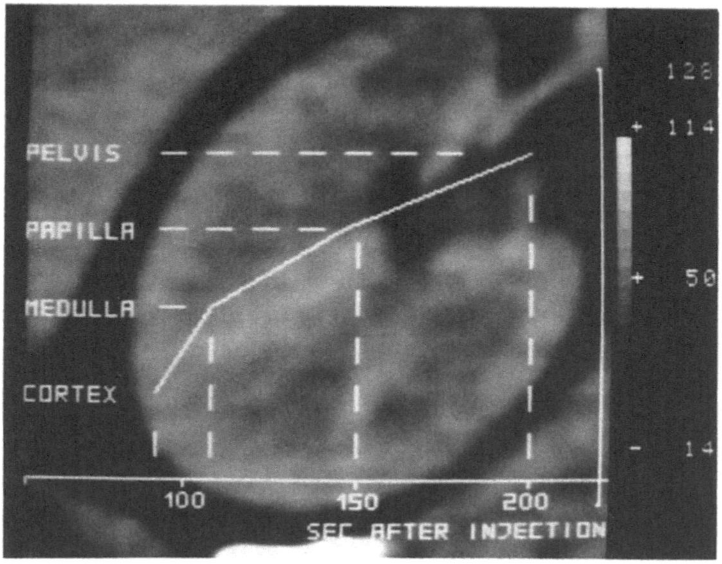

Fig. 10. Temporal sequence of filtration and excretion of contrast medium. Mean arrival times of the maximum enhancement are plotted for different areas of the kidney (normal renal function)

The temporal sequence of the filtration of contrast medium and the excretion of contrast urine into the renal pelvis can be demonstrated by plotting on a graph the arrival times of the maximum density values in the different parts of the kidney (Fig. 10).

Left and right kidneys were compared in 18 subjects with normal circulatory parameters and renal function, using the density values after injection of contrast medium and the resulting time-density curves for abdominal aorta and renal cortex, medulla, papilla, and pelvis. The shape and measured values were found to be similar in all cases. Enhancement curves of the healthy kidney obtained by other authors, e.g., *Hübener* and *Klott* (1980) and *Ishikawa* et al. (1981), are comparable in their qualitative tendencies with our findings. This correlation permits such results to be used as a standard for comparison.

4.2 Pathologic Findings

To study perfusion and excretion in renal insufficiency, 29 cases of renovascular hypertension were investigated using sequential CT. Two groups were selected – 20 patients suffering from hydronephrosis, and nine patients with a stenosis of the renal artery on one side. All cases had been checked clinically by renal scintigraphy or angiography.

4.2.1 Hydronephrosis

The enhancement curves varied according to the individual circulation parameters and degree of renal insufficiency. However, typical differences in the shape of the density curves in comparison to the normally functioning kidney on the healthy side can be described (Fig. 11, Fig. 13 curve 4).

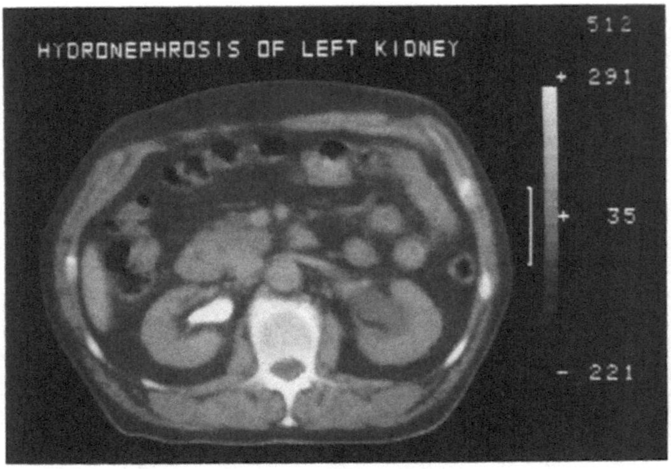

a

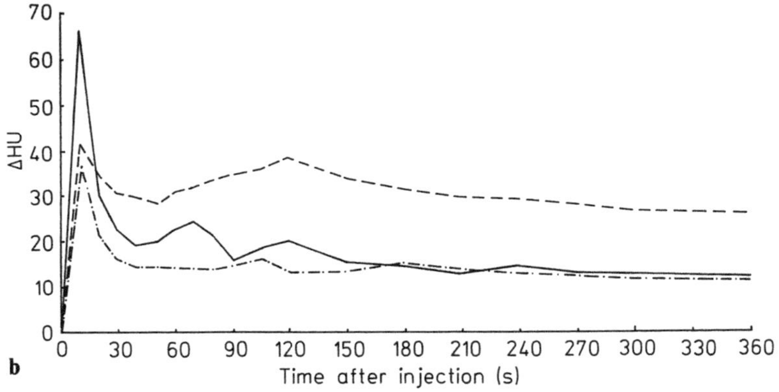

b

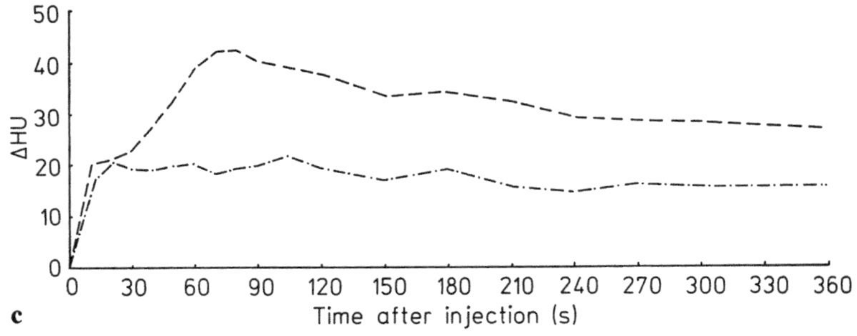

c

Fig. 11. a Scan level through the kidneys for a sequential CT investigation of a 51 year old patient suffering from hydronephrosis of the left kidney. For corresponding time-density curves see Fig. 11 b. **b, c** Enhancement curves for renal cortex (**b**) and medulla (**c**). The curves are typical for patients with hypertension due to hydronephrosis (see also Fig. 13). ——, abdominal aorta; – – – –, R cortex/medulla; –·–·– , L cortex/medulla

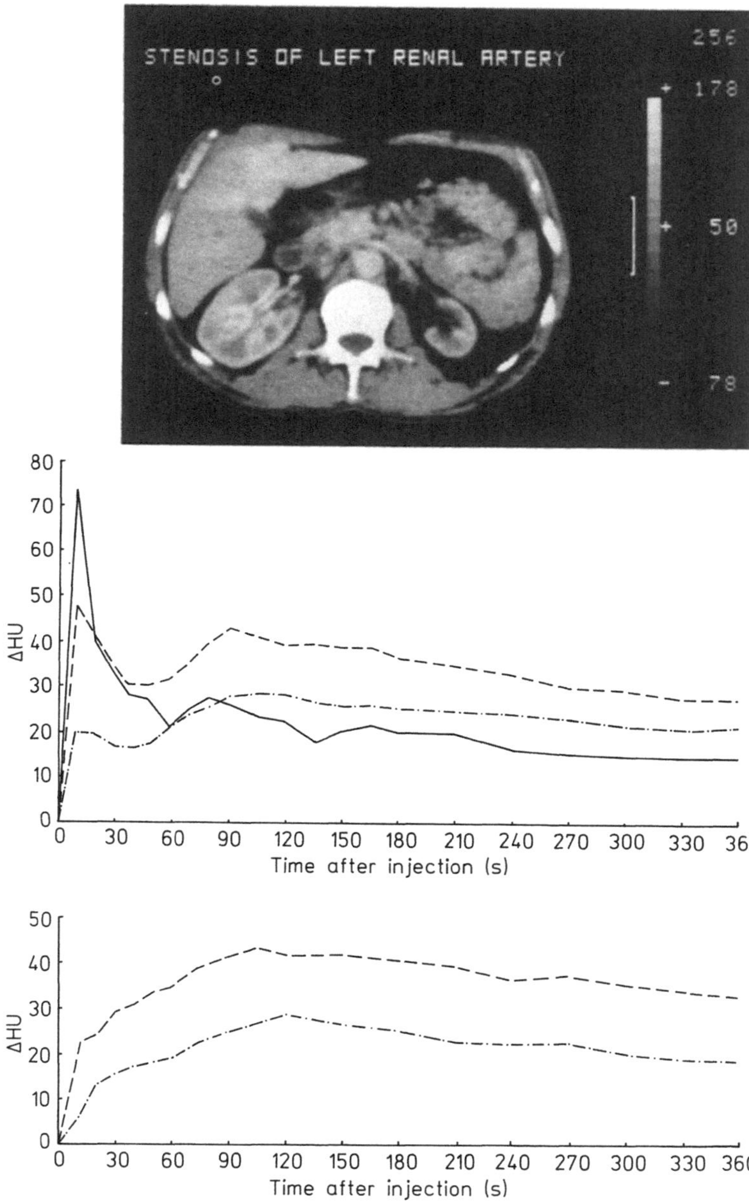

Fig. 12a–c. Sequential CT investigation of a 46-year-old patient with hypertension caused by stenosis of the left renal artery. **a** Scan through the kidneys. **b, c** Time-density curves for renal cortex (**b**) and medulla (**c**). Only low enhancement could be observed in the left renal pelvis of this patient – the kidney's contribution to urine excretion is drastically reduced. The curves can be generalized to patients suffering from hypertension due to stenosis of the renal artery (See also Fig. 13). ——, abdominal aorta; – – – –, R cortex/medulla; –·–·– , L cortex/medulla

Renal Cortex. The swift increase in density is similar to the enhancement observed in normal kidneys. The decrease which follows the initial enhancement peak is more rapid and no or only a slight secondary increase in density is observed, depending on the residual blood filtration capability of the kidney. If the kidney has lost this capability entirely, the enhancement in the cortex of the damaged kidney is determined by the filtration rate on the healthy side. In this case, the enhancement is as measured in the aorta.

Renal Medulla. The enhancement corresponds to that in the renal cortex. An increase in density is related to the remaining blood filtration capability. If this has been completely destroyed, the supply of the renal parenchyma with blood leads to enhancement reflecting the level of iodine in the aorta.

In the calices of a damaged kidney, as in the pelvis, enhancement corresponds to the residual filtration capability.

4.2.2 Renal Artery Stenosis

Typical patterns can also be established for time-density curves in stenosis of the renal artery (Fig. 12, Fig. 13 curve 3).

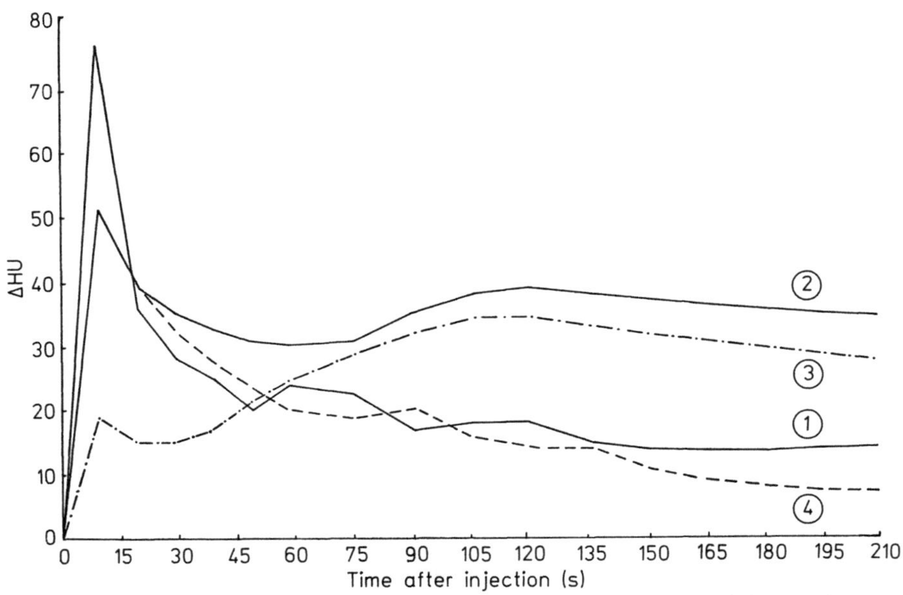

Fig. 13. Generalized time-density distribution in the abdominal aorta and the renal cortex after standard injection of contrast medium (30 ml, 300 mg iodine/ml, 6 ml/s) into the cubital vein. *1* The time-density curve for the aorta is plotted as a reference representing the input function of the excretory system. *2* Enhancement in the normal cortex. After an initial peak, a second increase in density due to the filtration of the opacified blood is observed. *3* Enhancement in the cortex of patients with hypertension due to stenosis of a renal artery. Depending on the degree of the stenosis, the initial enhancement peak is reduced in amplitude or is no longer observable. *4* Enhancement in the cortex of patients with hypertension due to hydronephrosis. After the typical initial peak, a second rise in density depends on the residual capacity of the kidney to filtrate the inflowing blood

Renal Cortex. The initial enhancement due to the first passage of the injected contrast medium bolus depends on the degree of stenosis. The amplitude of this initial enhancement peak is not as great as on the normal side, and no peak at all can be observed in the case of severe stenosis. The maximum value of the secondary enhancement due to filtration is later and lower than on the normal side. Because of the stenosis, less blood is delivered and thus less contrast medium can be filtered.

Renal Medulla. Initial enhancement is delayed as in the cortex, and maximum enhancement is reached later than on the normal side. As the parenchyma is not damaged, the filtration capacity of the kidney is not reduced, but owing to the decrease in blood supply, depending on the degree of stenosis, less blood is filtered. Thus enhancement in the medulla is less than in the case of normal renal blood supply.

The excretion of contrast urine from the calices to the pelvis is slower than on the normal side. The gradient of the enhancement is not as steep and the maximum density not as distinct as normal. In the case of total stenosis, no enhancement is observed. These findings are in correspondence with the results obtained by *Walz* et al. (1982) when studying the enhancement of healthy and damaged minipig kidneys.

5 Discussion

Sequential bolus CT enables not only morphological and vascular findings, but also functional diagnosis. The examination shows the different phases of perfusion with the possibility of simultaneous quantification. Pathologic processes can be imaged in different phases of perfusion and can therefore be used in differential diagnosis.

The additional importance of time-density curves for diagnosis becomes evident when visual differentiation and objectivation of unknown morphological structures or functional changes have not been possible with normal CT scanning. Thus bolus CT is helpful in evaluating the perfusion of the kidneys, especially in diseases like renal vascular stenosis with great variations in perfusion.

Dynamic CT studies of the kidneys can be used as a non-interventional method of screening patients suffering from renovascular hypertension. After standardized intravenous bolus injection of contrast medium, the time-density curves evaluated for the different kidney areas reflect the organ's function and the kinetics of the contrast medium used. The disadvantage of all sequential CT investigations is that perfusion studies can only be performed within a single 8-mm-thick preselected slice and are associated with a relatively high regional surface dose (18 mGy/scan). If the organ under investigation takes part in respiratory movement, care has to be taken that all images within a series are exposed in the same phase of the respiratory cycle, e.g., during expiration (*Reiser* 1980). Nevertheless, the results of an accurately undertaken investigation allow conclusions to be drawn concerning the blood circulation through the kidney and the general function of the organ. The time-density curves for the renal cortex and medulla provide – when compared to the curve for the aorta as the input function to the excretory system – more information about loss of function. Thus it can be determined whether a reduction in function is related to a structural lesion of the renal parenchyma, a hemodynamically significant stenosis of the renal artery, or a partial or total infarct.

The value of a very rapid, early starting series of images becomes especially evident when it is of importance to examine the vascular phase of perfusion, in which it is possible to use the enhancement in the extravascular space to recognize pathologic structures of the parenchyma and differentiate them from normal tissue. The administration of the contrast medium in the form of an injection or infusion in normal CT scanning could cause pathologic isodense areas to "disappear", and in this case the vascular phase could not be imaged unless the injection had by chance been made at the correct stage of exponation.

Standardization of the contrast medium bolus injection is essential if hemodynamic tendencies and types of curves are to be compared and related to specific clinical findings. Furthermore, a standard injection is required to define parameters for the concentration and excretion potential of the kidneys if a quantitative determination of renal function is desired. The potential of sequential CT scanning to quantify changes in contrast medium concentration after intravenous bolus injection means that it is applicable not only to the study of renovascular hypertension, as described, but also to a wide variety of other diseases.

The range of applications of sequential CT embraces those of other radiological procedures such as angiography, static CT, and nuclear medicine with the help of special image-processing programs. The advantages of sequential CT can be compressed into three points: (a) native, diagnostically obscure anatomical structures can be defined better; (b) pathologic processes can be imaged in different phases of perfusion and can thus be clarified by differential diagnosis; and (c) it becomes possible to draw conclusions on the function of the organ on the basis of its perfusion. The introduction of the sequential examination widens the diagnostic possibilities of CT.

6 Summary

As a dynamic investigation mode, sequential CT extends the possibilities of diagnostic radiology. Densitometric studies of the normal and pathologic kinetics of renal blood flow were carried out after intravenous bolus injection of renal contrast medium containing iodine. In comparative studies, the influence of the mode of injection (contrast medium flow, volume, and concentration) on the enhancement in the abdominal aorta was investigated to define standards. Time-density curves computed after standard injection of contrast medium into the cubital vein (30 ml, 300 mg iodine/ml, 6 ml/s) were evaluated for the different areas of the kidneys, such as the cortex and medulla. These curves permit conclusions to be drawn about the perfusion and correct function of the organ. Dynamic densitometric studies can help to detect the causes of renovascular hypertension (e.g., stenosis of the renal artery) and reduced renal filtration (e.g., hydronephrosis).

References

Axel L (1980) Cerebral blood flow determination by rapid-sequence computed tomography. Radiology 137:679–686

Baert AL, Wilms G, Marchal G, DeMayer P, DeSomer F (1980) Contrast enhancement by bolus technique in the CT examination of the kidney. Radiologe 20:279–287

Brennan RE, Curtis JA, Pollack HM, Weinberg I (1979a) Sequential changes in the CT numbers of the normal canine kidney following intravenous contrast administration. I. The renal cortex. Invest Radiol 14:141–148

Brennan RE, Curtis JA, Pollack HM, Weinberg I (1979b) Sequential changes in the CT numbers of the normal canine kidney following intravenous contrast administration. II. The renal medulla. Invest Radiol 14:239–245

Burgener FA, Hamlin DJ (1981) Contrast enhancement in abdominal CT: bolus vs. infusion. AJR 137:351–358

Decker D, Faust U, Reiser U (1983) Model experiments for angiocinedensitometry. In: Heuck FHW (ed) Radiological functional analysis of the vascular system. Springer, Berlin Heidelberg New York Tokyo

Fuchs WA, Vock P, Haertel M (1979) Pharmakokinetik intravasaler Kontrastmittel bei der Computer-Tomographie. Radiologe 19:90–93

Gardeur D, Lantrou J, Millard JC, Berger N, Metzger J (1980) Pharmacokinetics of contrast media: experimental results in dog and man with CT implications. J Comput Assist Tomogr 4:178–185

Heinz ER, Dubois PJ, Drayer BP, Hill R (1980) A preliminary investigation of the role of dynamic computed tomography in renovascular hypertension. J Comput Assist Tomogr 4:63–66

Heller M, Grabbe E, Bücheler E (1981a) Serien-Computertomographie – Methodik und erste Erfahrungen. Fortschr Röntgenstr 134:16

Heller M, Huland H, Hagemann J, Bischoff K (1981b) Computertomographische Diagnostik von renalen und extrarenalen Komplikationen bei Nierentransplantation – „statische" und „dynamische" Untersuchungen. Computertomographie 1:184–192

Hübener KH (1978) Computertomographische Densitometrie von Leber, Milz und Nieren bei intravenös verabreichten lebergängigen Kontrastmitteln in Bolusform. Fortschr Röntgenstr 129:289–297

Hübener KH, Klott KJ (1980) „Statisches" und dynamisches Kontrastmittelenhancement der Körperstamm-Computertomographie (Ortsauflösung, Angio-CT, Sequenz-CT). Fortschr Röntgenstr 133:347

Ishikawa I, Onouchi Z, Saito Y, Kitada H et al. (1981) Renal cortex visualization and analysis of dynamic CT curves of the kidney. J Comput Assist Tomogr 5:695–701

Ono N, Martinez CR, Fara JW, Hodges FJ (1980) Diatrizoate distribution in dogs as a function of administration rate and time following intravenous injection. J Comput Assist Tomogr 4:174–177

Reiser U, Heuck F, Pfeiler M (1980) Einfluß auf Quantifizierung der Atemverschieblichkeit von abdominellen Organen bei der Röntgencomputertomographie. Fortschr Röntgenstr 133:1; 9–17

Schad N, Schepke P, Rohde U, Schepke H, Schmid V, Breit A (1981) Timing of exposure in angiographic computed tomography. Cardiovasc Intervent Radiol 4:59–65

Walz PH, Klose K, Goldmann F, Evers E, Alken P (1982) Kontrastmittelabhängige Dichteveränderungen gesunder und geschädigter Nieren in der Sequenz-Computertomographie. Aktuel Urologie 13:33–36

Young SW, Noon MA, Nassi M, Castellino RA (1980) Dynamic computed tomography body scanning. J Comput Assist Tomogr 4:168–173

Percutaneous Transhepatic Drainage: Technique, Results, and Special Applications

R. Köster[1]

1 Strahleninstitut und Radiologische Klinik, Krankenanstalten Neuss, Lukaskrankenhaus, Akademisches Lehrkrankenhaus der Universität Düsseldorf, Preußenstr. 84, D-4040 Neuss.
Submitted for publication in April 1983

1 Introduction

Extrahepatic biliary surgery, including surgery of the papilla and gallbladder, has made great advances in recent decades. All the same, long-term success rates in the treatment of malignant obstructive jaundice are little better than 50 years ago, so that even today biliary tract and gallbladder carcinoma continues to have one of the worst prognoses amongst malignant tumours of the digestive tract. The reasons for this lie partly in the uncharacteristic symptomatology of these malignancies, which allows an early diagnosis in only a few cases, and partly in the high grade of the malignancy.

As the main symptoms are atypical upper abdominal pain and digestive complaints, most patients do not present for diagnostic assessment until jaundice has appeared. As a rule, this occurs late in biliary tract and gallbladder carcinomas, when extensive tumour or metastatic growth has already taken place. With carcinoma of the papilla, jaundice occurs earlier but is often intermittent, which delays the diagnosis. Recently developed methods of investigation such as ultrasonography and computer tomography (CT) have not led to earlier diagnosis of these malignancies. As long as no means of early diagnosis has been developed no improvement can be expected in the results of surgery.

With the introduction of percutaneous transhepatic biliary drainage it became possible for radiologists to make a better diagnostic assessment of obstructive jaundice and also to relieve biliary obstruction on a temporary or long-term basis.

This volume is concerned with the current status of percutaneous transhepatic cholangiography (PTC) and percutaneous transhepatic drainage (PTD) in the diagnosis and treatment of malignant and benign obstructive jaundice and the options for therapy that have arisen from these techniques. In particular, the influence of PTD on current surgical procedures and the development of a small-volume, high-dose form of radiotherapy based on an afterloading technique are described. In addition, the effect of intrahepatic biliary congestion on the portal circulation is demonstrated and discussed.

2 Recent Surgical Procedures in Obstructive Jaundice

Until recently once the diagnosis of obstructive jaundice was settled the next step was laparotomy, regardless of whether the cause was assumed to be benign or malignant. The decision regarding the ensuing operative procedure was left until after laparotomy. With malignant processes the procedure selected depends mainly on whether or not a biliodigestive anastomosis can be constructed.

The prerequisite for biliodigestive anastomosis (choledochojejunostomy, choledochoduodenostomy, hepaticojejunostomy) is a sufficiently long hepatic biliary duct. In a favourable case with a small tumour a radical operation (e.g., *Whipple's* operation) can be performed (Fig. 1). The decision to construct the high biliodigestive anastomosis in the perihilar region of the liver or an intrahepatic hepatodigestive anastomosis is taken only in isolated cases with smaller, easily resectable tumours when the patient's general condition is good and there are no metastases (*Corlette* and *Bookwalter* 1980).

A biliodigestive anastomosis can no longer be entertained when the tumour is extensive, especially with a tumour situated high up near the hepatic ducts or near the bifurcation of the hepatic duct (Fig. 2) or when several malignant strictures exist (Fig. 3). There are several different palliative operative procedures to choose from for bypassing the obstruction through the tumour.

Kehr T Drain (*Bünte* 1977; *Dittel* et al. 1978). After dilatation of the stricture in the tumour-bearing part, a T drain is inserted in such a manner that the centrally direct-

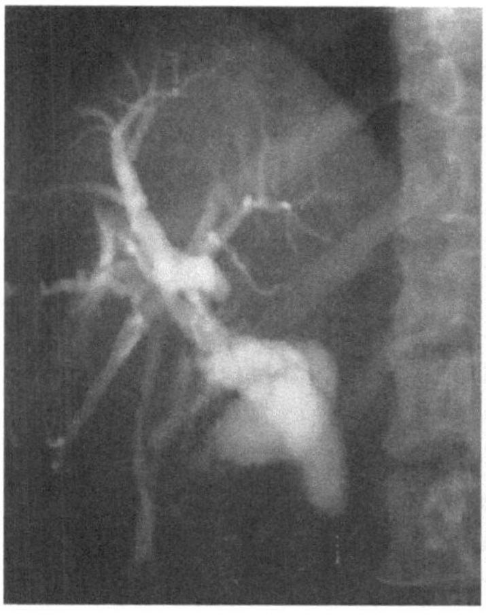

Fig. 1

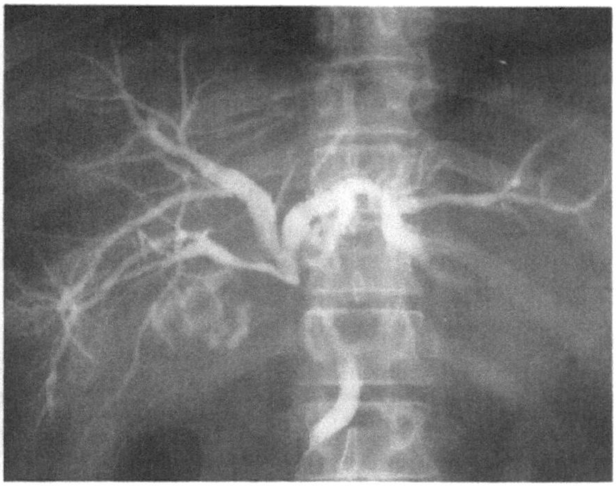

Fig. 2

Fig. 1. Carcinoma of the head of pancreas 8 mm in diameter in a 50-year-old female patient. Obstruction in the distal common bile duct and a small tumour indicate radical resection (Whipple's operation)

Fig. 2. Extensive gallbladder carcinoma infiltrating the hepatoduodenal ligament across to the bifurcation of the hepatic bile duct in a 46-year-old male patient. The extensive tumour growth combined with high localisation renders this patient unsuitable for a biliodigestive anastomosis

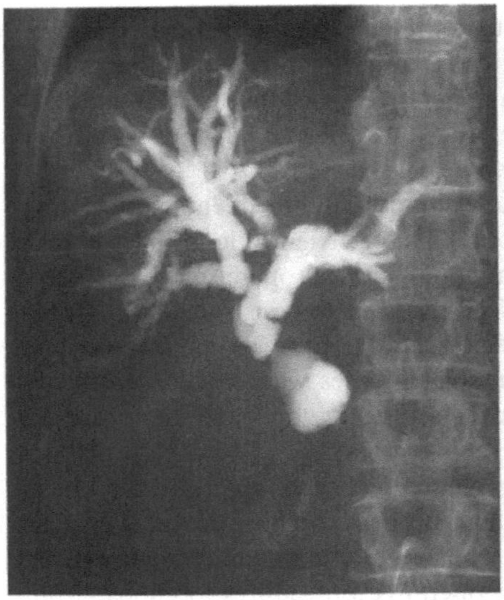

Fig. 3

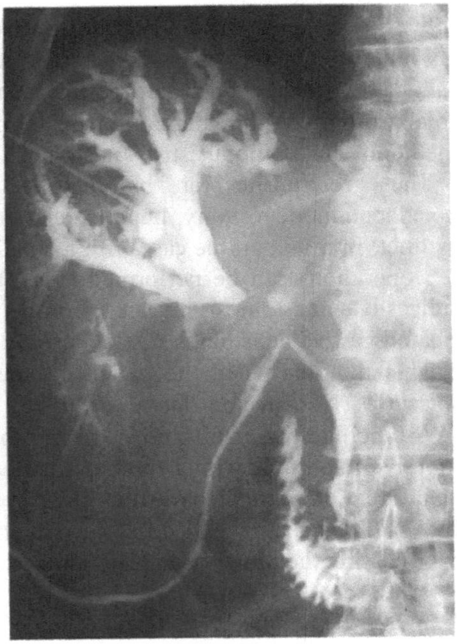

Fig. 4

Fig. 3. Distal obliteration of the common bile duct caused by carcinoma of the head of pancreas in a 67-year-old female patient. The stricture in the proximal hepatic bile duct due to additional metastases means that a biliodigestive anastomosis is no longer possible

Fig. 4. Inoperable bile duct carcinoma in a 73-year-old patient. Operative palliative procedure in the form of a Kehr T drain. Tumour spread has caused obliteration of the proximal limb of the T drain, which has ceased to function

ed branch lies in the bifurcation of the hepatic ducts. The main disadvantages of this type of drain are the easy obliteration by pressure exerted by the tumour (Fig. 4) and a tendency to encrust.

"Lost Drain" (*Black* et al. 1971). A silicon drain of roughly the thickness of a pencil and with numerous holes on the side is pushed through the dilated neoplastic stricture in the bile duct up to the bifurcation of the hepatic biliary ducts and left as an indwelling drain. *Peabody* and *Milimann* (1972) used a small vitallium tube in the same way as the silicon drain. These indwelling drains have the disadvantage that they may lose their function relatively soon through crust formation; furthermore, inadequate fixation makes it possible for them to perforate the duodenal wall (*Heim* and *Cramer* 1960).

Hartenbach Endoprosthesis (*Hartenbach* 1977). This is a lost drain in the form of a two-piece metal prosthesis that resists the tumour pressure for a long time and can be temporarily connected with the outside by tubing for flushing as with the Kehr drain (Fig. 5).

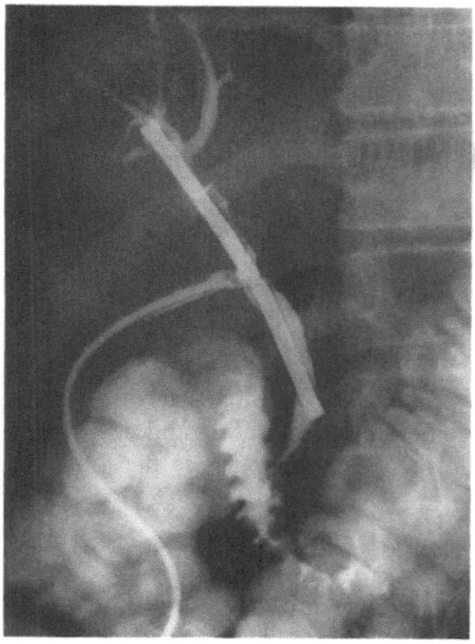

Fig. 5

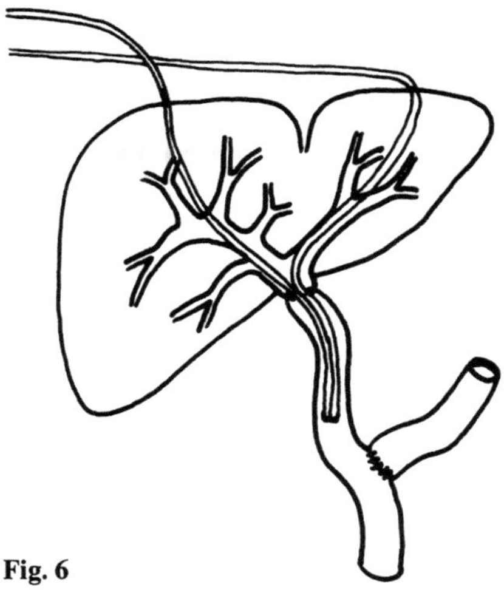

Fig. 6

Fig. 5. Inoperable, highly differentiated bile duct carcinoma in a 57-year-old patient. Palliative operation in the form of a Hartenbach bile duct endoprosthesis: a metal prosthesis in two parts connected to the exterior via a temporary tube facilitating regular washouts. The proximal end of the Hartenbach prosthesis is sited rather unfavourably high in the region of the right hepatic bile duct

Fig. 6. Rodney-Smith drainage. Palliative operation in the form of a hepaticojejunostomy with a tube lying in each of the right and left branches of the hepatic bile duct draining the anastomosed loop of the small bowel via the liver to the exterior

Smith Drain (*Smith* 1964). In the presence of a high bile duct obstruction a hepaticojejunostomy is constructed and drainage tubing inserted from the anastomosed loop of small bowel through both the right and left hepatic ducts through the liver draining to the outside (Fig. 6). The advantage of this method lies in the possibility of constant flushing of the system, thus preventing encrustation.

"U Tube" (*Terblanche* and *Lower* 1973; *Terblanche* et al. 1972). The U tube is a further development of the Smith drain, whereby in place of two separate drains a single drain in the form of a U leads from the exterior through the liver into the biliary tract, through the stricture and back to the outside. This method offers the advantage of easy replacement (without reoperation) in the event of encrustation.

Transhepatic Endless Drain (*Dick* and *Dortenmann* 1965; *Goetze* 1951; *Strunck* et al. 1979; *Heydenrych* et al. 1969). In principle, this is a similar drainage method to that with the U tube, but with a different route for the drains through the liver and adjacent anastomosed parts of the bowel. *Spieler* et al. (1977) closes the two free limbs of the endless drain subcutaneously to avoid any danger of infection from the outside. The drains are always accessible for flushing and changing by way of a small operative procedure performed under a local anaesthetic.

In the presence of extensive tumour growth none of the operative procedures described above can be performed, and the operation has to be completed in the form of an exploratory laparotomy. According to *Neugebauer* et al. (1979), the number of patients for whom the only option was an exploratory laparotomy was in the region of 40% for gallbladder carcinomas and about 30% for bile duct carcinomas.

3 Diagnostic Techniques in Obstructive Jaundice

Owing to a higher operative risk for jaundice patients, a decision regarding operability and choice of procedure should be made before the operation and not have to wait until the exploratory laparotomy is performed. For this purpose the following questions need to be answered:

1. Is the cause of jaundice "medical" or "surgical"?
2. At what level of the descending biliary ducts does the obstruction lie?
3. How extensive is the obstructive tumour; are metastases present?
4. Is the cause of bile duct obstruction benign or malignant?

The methods available for investigation vary in their usefulness: History, clinical examination of the patient, and laboratory investigations are of only very limited value for differentiation between surgical and medical jaundice. An increase of alkaline phosphatase with normal values for serum transaminases tends to indicate extrahepatic obstructive jaundice, but unfortunately nonspecific constellation of these values is found in up to 40% of patients (*Stern* et al. 1973).

Barium contrast studies of the stomach and duodenum show characteristic radiological signs, consisting in prestenotic dilatation of the bile ducts with displacement of the lateral duodenal wall by a hydropic gallbladder, a band-like impression in the duodenal bulb caused by dilated bile duct (*Riegel's* sign), and a droplet-shaped impression in the medial wall of the duodenum near the papilla (congestive impression due to a dilated common bile duct). Additional information regarding the causes of obstructive jaundice may be gained by these methods in cases in which a process involving the head of the pancreas has caused displacement or narrowing of the descending part of the duodenum or has lifted the duodenal bulb, or when a tumour of the pancreas or gallbladder has grown into the duodenum causing ulcerations through necrosis, or a papillary tumour has grown into the lumen of the duodenum.

Intravenous (indirect) cholangiography is applicable in only very few cases, as with bilirubin levels above 2 mg%; the hepatic bile duct does not opacify at all, or only faintly, despite tomography and possibly even with continued infusion.

Cynn et al. (1979) recently demonstrated the use of infusion hepatotomography in the diagnosis of obstructive jaundice, whereby after administration of large volumes of contrast medium capable of renal passage the dilated intra- and extrahepatic biliary ducts are said to be demonstrable by negative contrast.

Liver scanning with the aid of radiolabelled colloids that are stored in the reticuloendothelial system (RES) only allows assessment of the size of the liver and the suspicion of larger space-occupying lesions near the hilus of the liver as well as of intrahepatic metastases.

A more valuable method for deciding whether the jaundice is obstructive or intrahepatic in origin in early cases is hepatobiliary sequence scintigraphy using radiolabelled substances capable of biliary passage: obstructions to bile flow can be demonstrated by this noninvasive method with bilirubin values up to 5 mg/100 ml (8 mg/100 ml at the most), even when the biliary system is not yet dilated or has been dilated in the past (e.g. after papillotomy).

The only sufficiently reliable noninvasive methods of differentiating between surgical and medical jaundice are those offered by ultrasound and CT, as these are not affected by the level of bilirubin or liver dysfunction. The correct diagnosis of obstructive jaundice can be obtained and the localisation of the obstruction determined equally well with either method (*Goldberg* et al. 1978): in up to 97% of cases with ultrasound (*Rettenmaier* 1977; *Sivaprasad* and *Gopalaswamy* 1980), and in up to 98% of patients with CT (*Havrilla* et al. 1977; *Levitt* et al. 1977; *Stanley* et al. 1977). It is possible to determine the aetiology of the obstruction in 62% by ultrasonography (*Rettenmaier* 1977), and in 72%–76% by CT (*Morris* et al. 1977; *Scherer* et al. 1979). In addition, both methods give valuable information regarding the extent of tumour growth and possible intrahepatic metastases.

After arriving at the diagnosis of obstructive jaundice by ultrasound or CT, precise identification of the obstructive lesion is necessary to allow an assessment of whether an anastomosing operation is possible. This can only be done by invasive means using direct cholangiography, either endoscopic retrograde cholangiography (ERC) or percutaneous transhepatic cholangiography (PTC).

ERC generally makes it possible to demonstrate the biliary system distal to the obstruction and proximal to the stenosis in the cases of incomplete obstruction. This, however, demands a great deal of endoscopic experience (*Bilbao* et al. 1976; *Katon* et al. 1974; *Nebel* and *Formes* 1973). The advantage of ERC over PTC lies in the additional endoscopic assessment of duodenum, papilla, and pancreas; the disadvantage is the risk of pancreatitis or rupture of pancreatic pseudocystes (*Sivaprasad* and *Gopalaswamy* 1980).

With PTC, the topographical and anatomical situation of the biliary duct system above the level of the obstruction can be visualised in almost all cases, which is extremely important for the planning of the operative procedure.

ERC and PTC are complementary methods; in cases where the ERC does not permit visualisation of the proximal end of the obstruction (Figs. 7 and 8) or where the procedure cannot be performed for technical reasons (e.g. in patients who have had anastomosing gastrointestinal operations, biliodigestive anastomoses, pyloric stenoses, or duodenal diverticula), PTC is definitely superior to ERC.

In view of the difficulty of assessing obstructive jaundice and the possibilities offered by the new noninvasive methods of investigation, such as ultrasound and CT, laparoscopy is no longer indicated (*Blumgart* 1976).

Angiography of visceral arteries now plays a minor role in the investigation of obstructive jaundice, although it is said to offer a high degree of accuracy in the case of common bile duct carcinoma, carcinoma of the papilla, and carcinoma of the head of the pancreas (*Olsson* and *Tylén* 1972) as well as providing, simultaneously, a direct method of visualising the biliary or pancreatic ducts (*Classen* et al. 1973; *Her-*

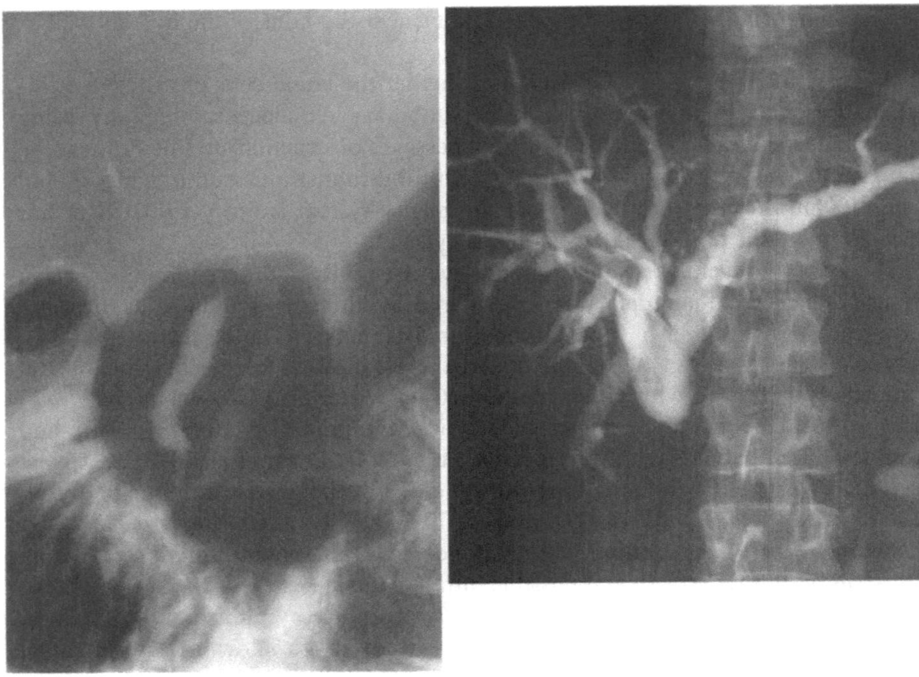

a b

Fig. 7 a, b. Metastases from a vaginal carcinoma to the hepatoduodenal ligament in a 50-year-old female patient. **a** ERCP shows fragmentation of the distal common bile duct just above the head of pancreas. Conclusions regarding the exact extent of the tumour obstructing the common bile duct cranially are not possible. **b** PTC shows a conical fragmentation of the severely congested hepatic bile duct where it meets the common bile duct. The length of the hepatic bile duct is adequate for an anastomosing operation

mann et al. 1974) and demonstrating liver metastases. In isolated cases preoperative angiography (arteriography *Suzuki* et al. 1980; *Tylen* et al. 1977), percutaneous transhepatic portography (*Hoevels* et al. 1983; *Popper* et al. 1954; *Reichart* and *Ihse* 1980), and CT or ultrasound can play a decisive role in the assessment of the possibilities and limitations of tumour surgery.

Given the availability of all investigative methods and considering the relative value of each method, the investigation of a case of jaundice (Fig. 9) should logically begin with the history and clinical examination of the patient and laboratory investigations. If haemolytic or hepatic cellular causes of jaundice have been excluded, the next stage is ultrasound or CT. Which of these two methods is used depends on the availability and on the examiner's experience, particularly in the case of ultrasound. If a congested biliary system is found, PTC or ERC, or if necessary both in combination, are performed to gain further information.

As a rule, these methods of investigation give the answers to all the questions raised in the assessment of operability and operative procedure.

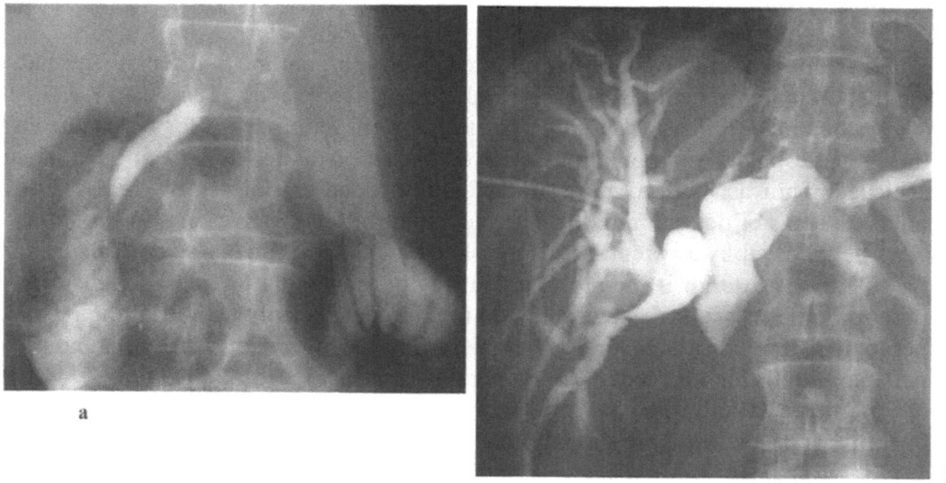

Fig. 8a, b. Bile duct carcinoma and central metastases in a 66-year-old female patient. **a** ERCP reveals a wide distal common bile duct with spindle-shaped cut-off at the level of L1. Opacification of the proximal part of the common bile duct is deficient. **b** PTC shows a spindle-shaped cut-off in the common hepatic bile duct immediately below the bifurcation in the presence of an obstructed intrahepatic biliary system. In this case, PTC reveals the high tumour obstruction in the common hepatic bile duct, which is unsuitable for a biliodigestive anastomosis

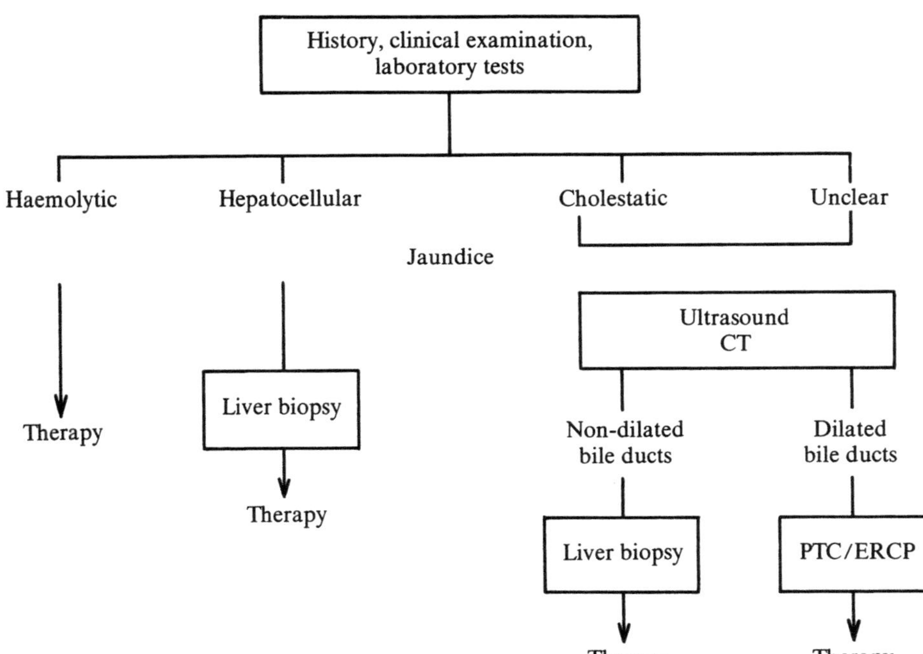

Fig. 9. Flow chart for differential diagnosis of obstructive jaundice

4 Indications for PTC and PTD

Whereas until recently PTC was considered the traditional method for differentiating between hepatocellular diseases and obstructive lesions (*Schütt* and *Köster* 1979), the dilated biliary tract is the most important requirement for percutaneous transhepatic biliary manipulations. The diagnosis of dilated biliary ducts is now achieved noninvasively and more simply by ultrasound or, if necessary, by CT. PTC offers a means of determining the site and extent of the obstruction and should always be followed by a percutaneous transhepatic biliary drainage, since drainage of the bile to the exterior is the most certain way of preventing the most serious complication of PTC, viz. leakage of bile into the peritoneal cavity with resulting biliary peritonitis. The indications for PTD arise from the high operative risk of jaundiced patients and the high percentage of inoperable cases (*Köster* et al. 1979).

The duration and degree of preoperative extrahepatic cholestasis and the postoperative mortality rate are directly related (*Coutsoftides* et al. 1977; *Fortner* et al. 1977; *Ihse* et al. 1977; *Maki* et al., 1966; *Mori* et al. 1977; *Nakase* et al. 1977; *Sato* et al. 1968). Patients with high serum bilirubin (over 20 mg%) have a mortality rate about twice as high as that for patients with slight jaundice (*Braasch* and *Gray* 1977; *Brooks* and *Culebras* 1976); postoperative mortality rates (defined as death occurring within 30 days of operation) quoted in the literature vary between 10% and 30% (*Coutsoftides* et al. 1977; *Feduska* et al. 1971; *Glen* and *Thorbjanarson* 1964; *Ihse* et al. 1977; *Maki* et al. 1966; *Morge* et al. 1964; *Nakase* et al. 1977; *Royer* et al. 1942; *Sato* et al. 1968; *Schmidt* et al. 1977; *Van Heerden* et al. 1967; *Warren* et al. 1962). For this reason a two-stage operation is often performed, in which the first step consists in institution of drainage, usually to the exterior (*Braasch* and *Gray* 1977; *Brooks* and *Culebras* 1976; *Catell* and *Pyrtek* 1949; *Hess* 1965; *Maki* et al. 1966; *Priestley* and *Wollaeger* 1961; *Rettenmaier* 1977; *Ross* 1959). Once decongestion of the biliary system and a fall in bilirubin level have been achieved, the patients suitable for radical resection undergo a second operation with a significantly lower operative risk. The improved operability can be attributed to the recovery of liver parenchyma, a decrease in bleeding tendency, amelioration of hypoproteinaemia, and improvement of the patient's nutritional state.

Even the first-stage decompression operation involves a considerable risk (*Buckwalter* et al. 1965; *Feduska* et al. 1971; *Hertzberg* 1974). It can be replaced by percutaneous transhepatic biliary drainage. *Takada* et al. (1976) published reports of an improvement in the mortality rate of tumour operations; the rate was reduced from 41% without decompression to less than 4% with decompression by means of biliary drainage. Improved mortality, reflected in reductions from 28.3% to 8.2% and even from 23% down to 0, has been reported by *Nakayama* et al. (1978) and *Rückert* et al. (1979), respectively. Biliary drainage has a great advantage over decompression operations, as it causes relatively little inconvenience to the patient (no operation and no anaesthetic), and demands relatively little in the way of personnel and expense. Additionally, during the second-stage operation the surgeon is unlikely to be confronted with operative difficulties caused by adhesions from the first decompression procedure.

The surgical alternatives are often very limited with malignant biliary duct obstructions: about 80%–90% of patients are already incurable by the time of operation (*Ferruci* et al. 1980), owing to the infiltration of tumour into adjacent organs or large vessels. In 30% of cases palliative anastomosis is no longer possible. The operative mortality rate after explorative laparotomy, with or without palliative biliodigestive anastomosis, may be as high as 30% (*Ferruci* et al. 1980). Patients with biliodigestive anastomosis tend to live 5–7 months longer than those without (*Bayindir* 1966; *Feduska* et al. 1971). Five-year survival rates are quoted at 6% as a maximum in cases of gallbladder carcinoma (*Dittel* et al. 1978) (80% of those with radical or palliative operation died after 1 year; without local procedures all patients were dead after 8 months (*Enderling* 1974), 5% in the case of carcinoma of the head, of the pancreas, 15% in periampullary carcinoma, and 25%–36% in purely papillary carcinoma (*Bedacht* and *von Bary* 1975/76; *Coutsoftides* et al. 1977; *Dittel* et al. 1978; *Kremer* et al. 1967).

A look at the poor life expectancy in these cases makes PTD definitely preferable to a decompression operation as a means of palliation (Figs. 10 and 11), particularly as improved survival is independent of the drainage method employed (intraoperative or nonoperative).

The lowered operative risk due to the reduction in bilirubin levels has resulted in the preoperative use of PTD in cases of benign obstructive jaundice such as that caused by stones (Fig. 12) or papillary stenoses (Fig. 13), and delaying operation until the bilirubin level has dropped. In addition, PTD may offer more diagnostic information than PTC alone: the indwelling catheter makes it simpler and safer to completely fill the biliary tree with contrast medium by altering the position of the patient. Significant findings besides a stone can be visualised before operation, thus reducing unforeseen intraoperative difficulties in a few cases (Figs. 14 and 15).

Benign strictures are also an indication for biliary drainage. Benign strictures of the hepatic bile duct are due to surgical lesions in 97% of cases (*Smith* 1964). Of all attempts at reconstructive surgery, which usually consist in or end in a hepaticojejunostomy, only 60% are successful. In the remaining 40% of cases the stenosis persists, with resulting recurrent ascending cholangitis, chronic hepatitis with pruritis, and possibly even portal hypertension. The operative mortality of these cases is around 13% (*Smith* 1964). PTD offers an alternative as a preoperative means of decompression, or even as long-term therapy in the form of internal drainage in the presence of very narrow strictures with little chance that surgery will be successful (Fig. 16). A further indication for PTD is postoperative splinting and relief of bile flow through the anastomosis to prevent anastomotic insufficiency (Fig. 17).

There are extremely few absolute contraindications for PTC with subsequent PTD: these include lack of patient cooperation, bleeding tendency irreversible by drugs, or parasitic diseases (*Echonococcus*). Prothrombin time (Quick) and thrombocyte counts are not decisive (*Göthlin* and *Transberg* 1973), as the coagulability of blood in the liver is not greatly influenced by a low Quick value. *Tylen* et al. (1977) quotes the lower limit for the Quick value as 30 and that for the thrombocyte count as 80,000, but he does not consider these as absolute limits. If necessary, vitamin K_1 infusions can be given before the PTD (*Ariyama* et al. 1978; *Nakayama* et al. 1978).

Acute suppurative cholangitis and even liver abscess are not contraindications for biliary drainage (Fig. 18): *Takada* et al. (1976) treated 16 patients, *Molnar* and *Stockum* (1974) one patient, and *Nakayama* et al. (1978) 11 patients with multiple

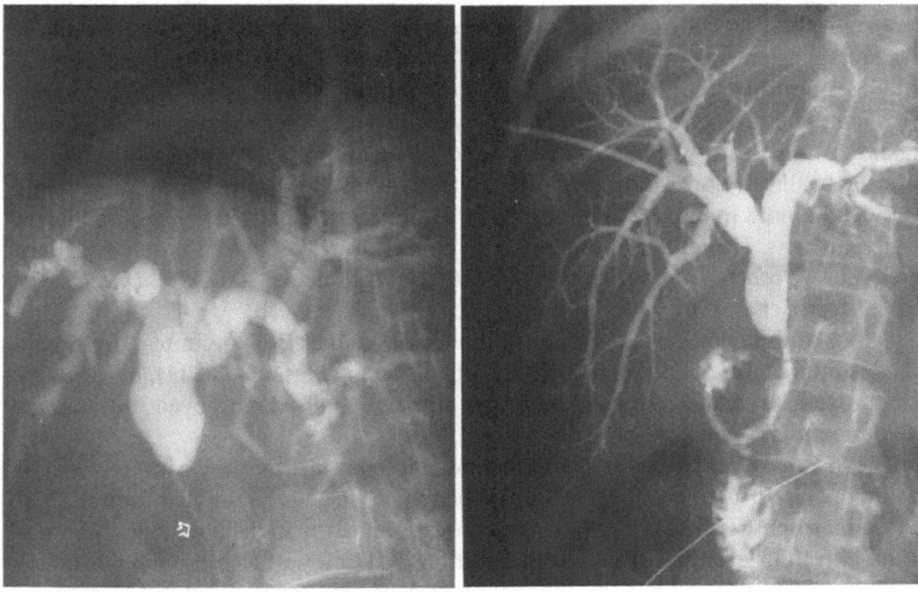

a, b

Fig. 10 a, b. Metastasising carcinoma of the head of the pancreas in a 58-year-old female patient. **a** PTC reveals thread-like stenosis of the intrahepatic common bile duct, with convexly limited cut-off in the maximally dilated common hepatic bile duct. **b** Internal drainage (PTD) was instituted, with the distal end of the catheter lying in the descending part of the duodenum

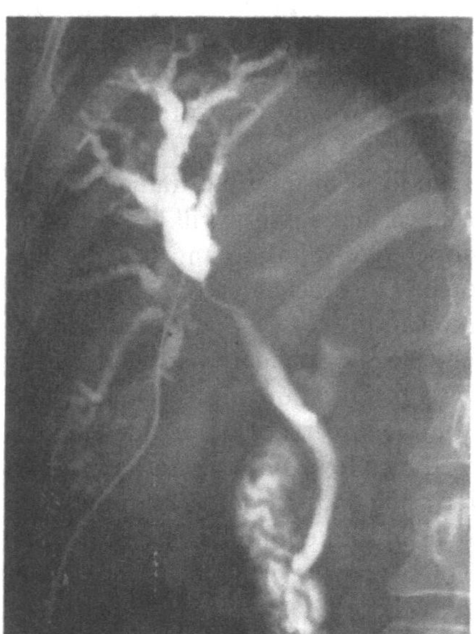

Fig. 11. Highly localised, inoperable biliary/hepatic bile duct carcinoma in a 57-year-old patient. A tight central stenosis is obstructing three intrahepatic biliary branches

Fig. 13 a, b. Sclerotic sphincter in a 85-year-old ▶ patient. **a** PTC reveals opacification of the maximally obstructed common hepatic bile duct with a conical prepapillary stenosing lesion with overflow of contrast medium into the duodenum. **b** For internal percutaneous transhepatic drainage the catheter has been inserted through the stenosis into the transverse part of the duodenum. (The patient refused surgery.)

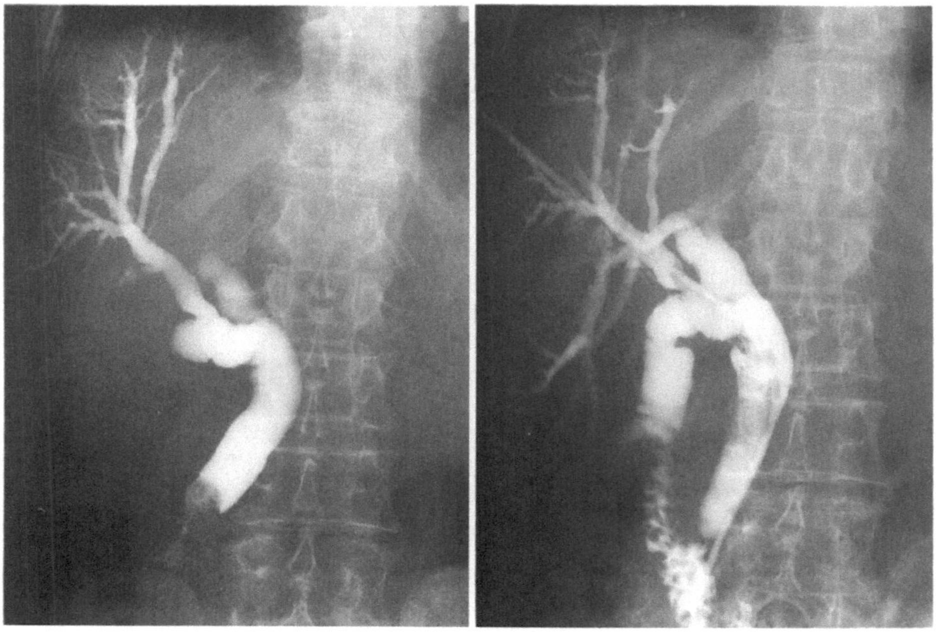

a b

Fig. 12a, b. Obstructive jaundice in a 74-year-old female patient. **a** PTC shows opacification of an obstructed intra- and extrahepatic biliary system with a filling defect suggestive of a concretion at least 2 cm in diameter in the distal common bile duct. **b** Internal percutaneous transhepatic drainage was instituted, and the filling defect now lies more distally in the hepatic bile duct which proves that a stone is the cause

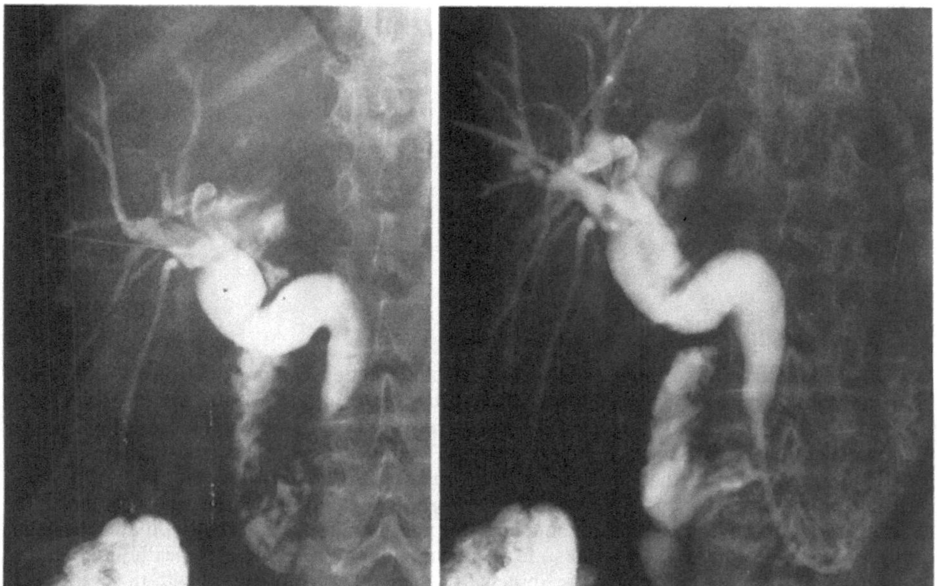

a b

Fig. 13a, b

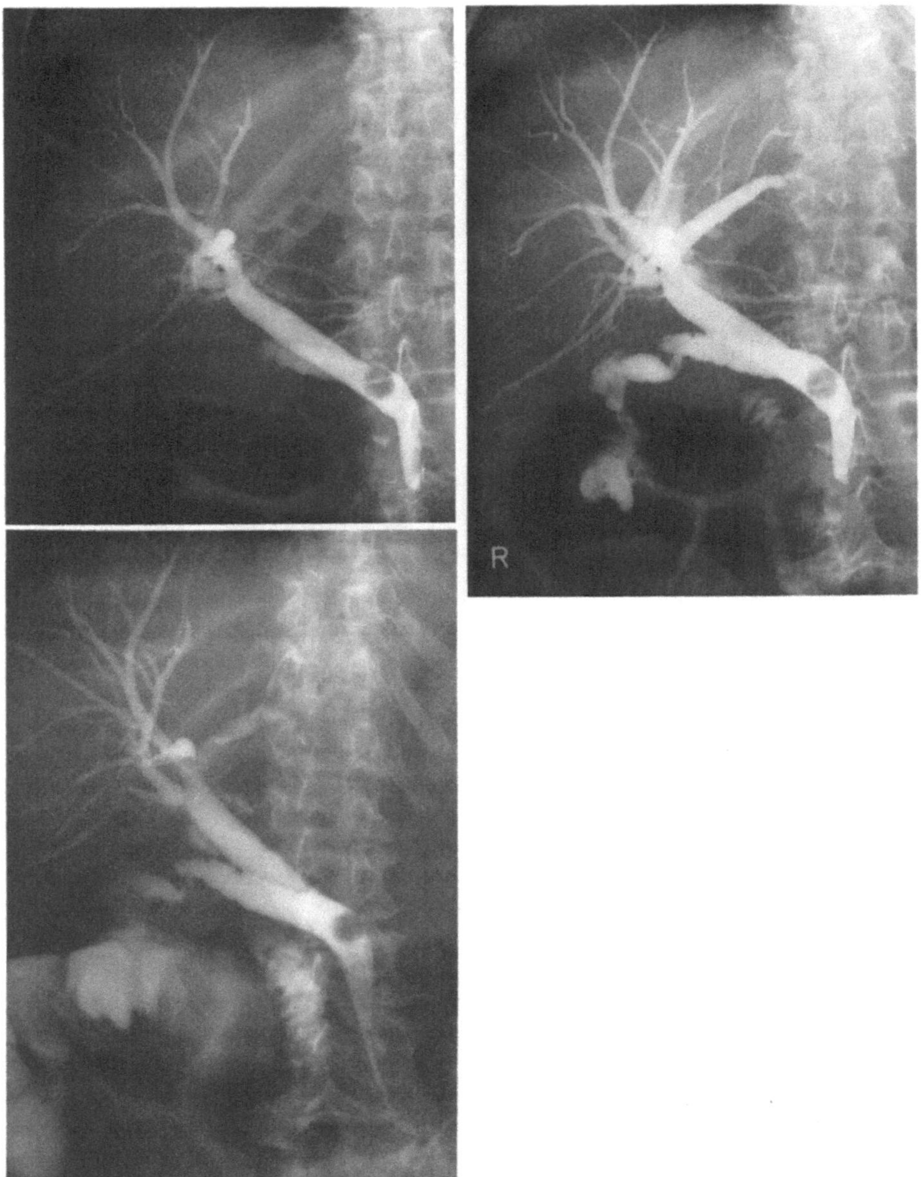

a b c

Fig. 14a–c. Obstructive jaundice in a 71-year-old female patient. Provisional diagnosis: malignant lesion. **a** PTC reveals an opacified obstructed common hepatic bile duct and partially filled cystic duct, also obstructed. A calculus at least 1 cm in diameter is lodged where the hepatic duct merges with the common bile duct. There is no flow of contrast medium into the duodenum. **b** After a further injection of contrast medium a subhepatic outflow of contrast medium from the cystic duct into an irregularly shaped cavity is demonstrable in the PTC, with a simultaneous flow of contrast medium through the papilla into the duodenum. **c** After insertion of an internal PTD it is possible to fill the biliary tree completely, without risk. Adequate opacification of the subhepatic abscess cavity, which communicates with the cystic duct as well as the right colonic flexure via a wide fistula channel, is now possible. The final diagnosis reached in this patient was obstructive jaundice due to choledocholithiasis and cystocolic fistula in the presence of calculus obstructing the cystic duct

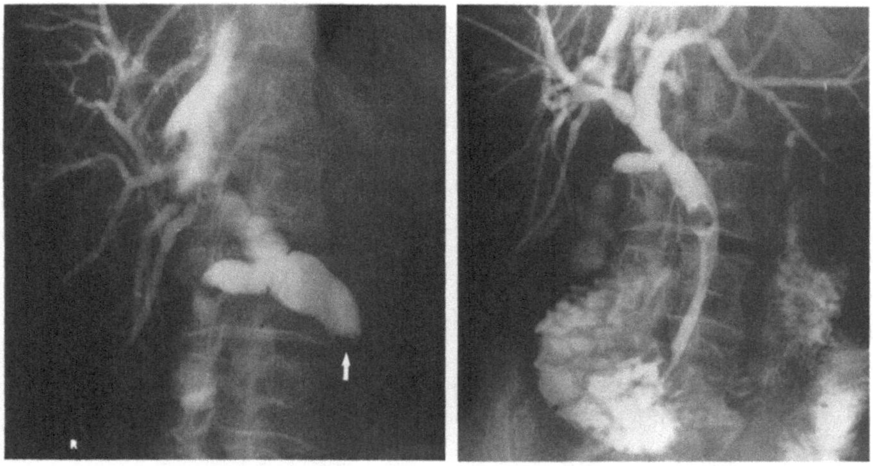

a b

Fig. 15a, b. Obstructive jaundice in a 63-year-old female patient. **a** PTC reveals a complete cut-off halfway up the common bile duct, with marked dilatation of the hepatic duct, intrahepatic biliary channels and cystic duct. The gallbladder cannot be adequately assessed. **b** For PTD the drainage catheter can be inserted through the obstructed common bile duct into the duodenum. Optimal contrast filling of the intra- and extrahepatic bile ducts allows visualisation of a large encrusted concretion in the common bile duct. Additionally, opacification of a small irregularly limited gallbladder (shrunken gallbladder with pericholecystitis/gallbladder carcinoma?) is seen

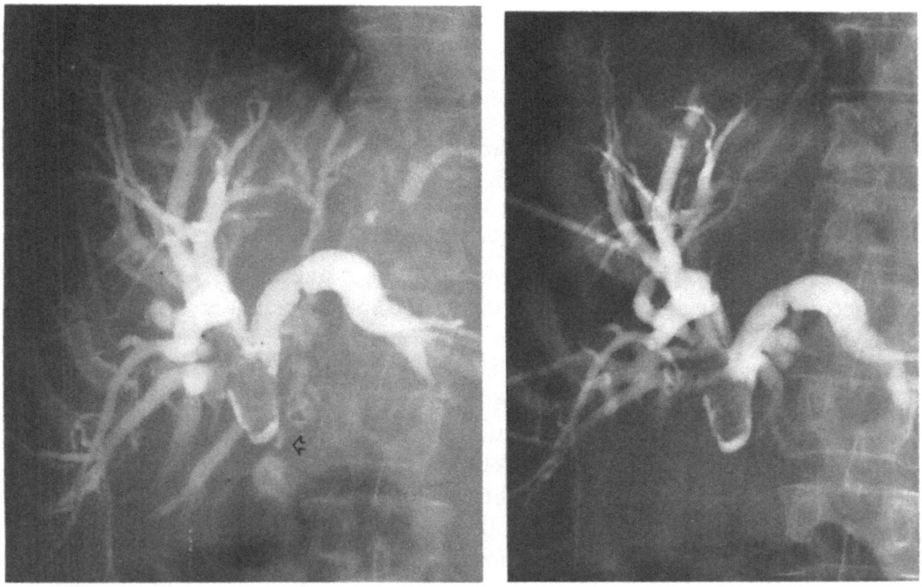

a b

Fig. 16a, b. Stricture in a hepaticojejunostomy in a 66-year-old patient. **a** PTC reveals the short stricture of the hepaticojejunostomy and a large biliary concretion obstructing the common hepatic bile duct. **b** External PTD was instituted; the catheter tip lies in the hepatic bifurcation distal to the calculus

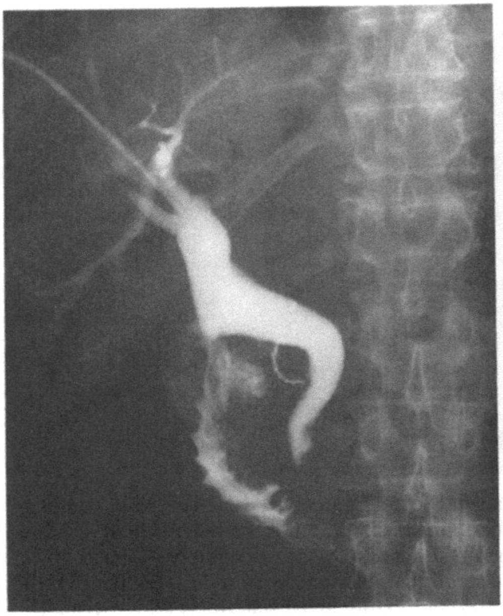

Fig. 17

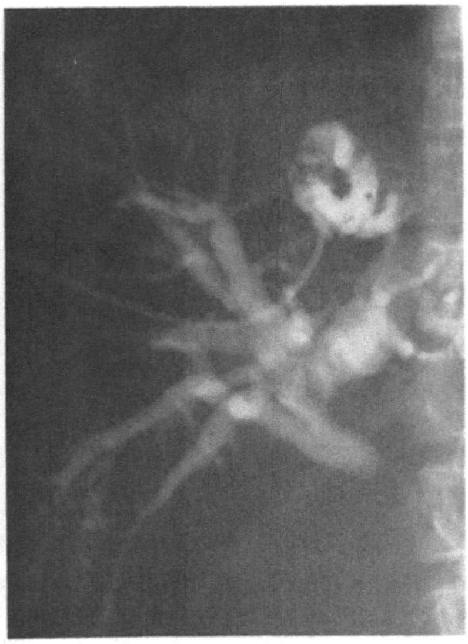

Fig. 18

Fig. 17. Obstructive jaundice due to carcinoma of the head of the pancreas in a 67-year-old patient. Postoperative findings after palliative choledochojejunostomy: temporary postoperative decompression of the anastomosis through an indwelling internal percutaneous drainage

Fig. 18. Carcinoma of the head of the pancreas in a 72-year-old female patient. Strong clinical suspicion of multiple liver abscesses. External drainage was instituted with the Catheter tip lying in a large abscess cavity and the side-holes in the obstructed region of the hepatic bile duct

intrahepatic gallstones and acute suppurative cholangitis. Of these patients, five had multiple intrahepatic abscesses. Immediate institution of biliary drainage with decompression of the biliary system and intensive washouts with salt solutions and antibiotics made the patients suitable for operation.

Poor general condition and ascites are not contraindications; on the contrary, the procedure may be all the more necessary in such circumstances.

Molnar and *Stockum* (1974) consider a normal renal function as a prerequisite for PTD and regard hepatorenal insufficiency as a contraindication. This opinion is based on the experience that significantly more patients with obstructive jaundice than without jaundice suffer acute renal failure in the postoperative phase (*Funck-Brentano* et al. 1963; *Williams* et al. 1960) and the prognosis of these postoperative renal failures is very poor, with mortality up to 69% (*Kennedy* et al. 1973). On the other hand, it is the jaundice that can be relieved by PTD, consequently reducing the increased rate of postoperative complications, so that simultaneous renal insufficiency really renders PTD more necessary. For reasons of safety one should, however, attempt to improve renal function by infusions of mannitol, according to the principles of pre-, intra-, and postoperative management suggested by *Dawson* (1965).

5 Technique of PTC and PTD

5.1 Historical Aspects

The history of transhepatic cholangiography began with lateral and transhepatic punctures of the gallbladder performed in animals and three patients by *Burckhardt* and *Muller* (1921). In postmortem studies the gallbladder and intra- and extrahepatic biliary system could be visualised after the injection of contrast medium, whereas in vivo only the gallbladder could be visualised.

A ventrally approached transperitoneal gallbladder puncture carried out during laparoscopy was described by *Royer* et al. and also by *Lee* in 1942. This technique is still used today, as it involves a very low complication rate of 0.3% when performed with meticulous care (*Wannagat* 1973, 1974); this method of biliary tract investigation is restricted, however, in that the cystic duct has to be patent to allow the hepatic duct to be filled with contrast medium (*Swart* et al. 1976).

Percutaneous transhepatic puncture of intrahepatic bile ducts to achieve diagnostic filling of the biliary system (PTC) was performed by *Huard* and *Do-Xuan-Hop* in 1937. Following the work of *Carter* and *Saypol* (1952) and of *Leger* et al. (1952) this method quickly gained a reputation.

Carter and Saypol approached the left lobe of the liver ventrally to puncture the biliary system of a 36-year-old patient with obstructive jaundice. After determination of the biliary cause of obstruction the catheter needle was left in situ ("the retained needle acting as an operative choledochostomy"). The patient died 7 days later, by which time the jaundice had faded considerably.

Leger, too, indicated the value of biliary decompression via PTC during preoperative preparation and the possibility of instilling antibiotics. Leger received heavy criticism from his teacher Caroli because of the excessively high risk this procedure involved.

Following this, PTC was introduced in numerous clinics and continued to be developed. Meanwhile a large number of positive experiences has been reported and accumulated. From German-speaking regions publications include those of *Peiper* et al. (1967), *Rüttimann* et al. (1965), *Wenz* (1967), *Bayindir* (1966, 1973), *Adolph* (1908), *Swart* (1968), *Schütt* and *Köster* (1970).

In recent years PTC has been significantly improved by the introduction of the fine-needle technique (Chiba needle) by *Otho* et al. (1973), *Okuda* et al. (1974) and *Ariyama* et al. (1978). Surprisingly, the authors of numerous publications contented themselves for a long time with the diagnostic aspects of bile flow obstruction. *Leger* et al. (1952) described percutaneous transhepatic biliary drainage as long ago as 1952, but this did not result in greater popularity. After performing PTC, *Özdemir* and *Lancaster* (1971) aspirated as much bile as possible from the congested biliary system. *Zinberg* et al. (1965) left the catheter in the biliary duct system after puncture for drainage until the operation, a method that was employed in many clinics (*Swart* et al. 1976) without being subsequently developed for bile duct drainage.

Ideas produced by *Okuda* et al. (1974) on the Japanese side and on the American side by *Molnar* and *Stockum* (1978) who, having performed drainage, used the method for temporary drainage in operable cases and as internal or external long-term drainage in inoperable cases, focussed attention on this method and paved the way for its widespread use and the development of several techniques (*Nakayama* et al. 1978; *Mori* et al. 1977; *Ukai* et al. 1971; *Takada* et al. 1976; *Hoevels* et al. 1978; *Tylén* et al. 1977; *Burcharth* and *Nielbo* 1976; *Ring* et al. 1978; *Günther* et al. 1979; *Köster* et al. 1979).

5.2 Technique

The first series of PTD procedures in our clinic was carried out in the form of three-stage catheterisation (Fig. 19).

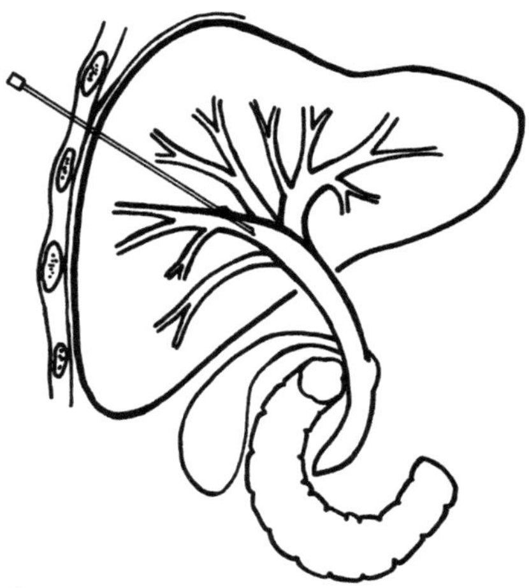

a

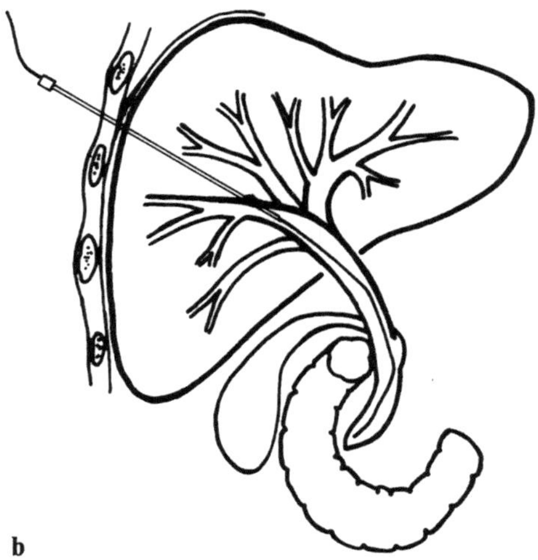

b

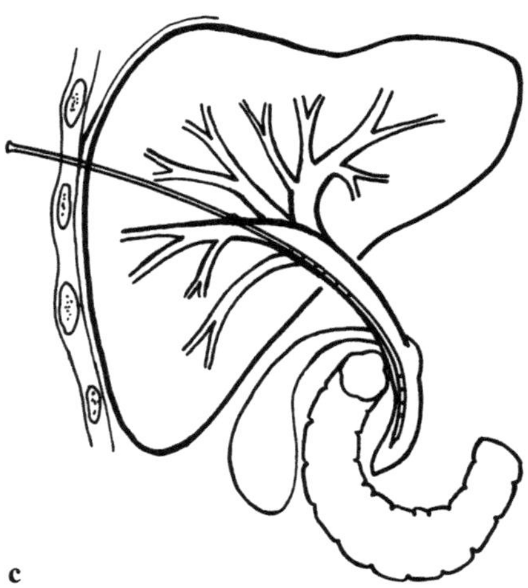

c

Fig. 19a–c. Diagram of the three-stage catheterisation technique for percutaneous transhepatic biliary drainage: **a** puncture with the Chiba needle for percutaneous transhepatic cholangiography; **b** puncture with the Teflon needle catheter for the introduction of the guide wire; **c** substitution (Seldinger technique), of an internal biliary drainage catheter (with the side-holes lying above and below the stenosis)

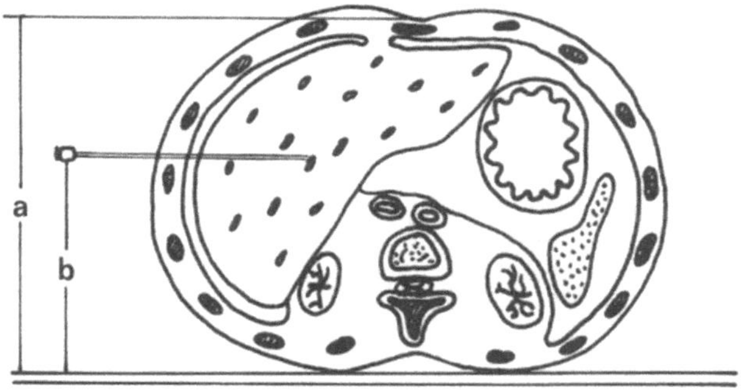

Fig. 20. Diagram of the direction of puncture in PTC in the transverse plane.

Table to sternum distance	Table to cannula distance
a = less than 19.5 cm	b = 11 cm
a = more than 19.5 cm	b = 12 cm

The first step is PTC using a Chiba needle to determine and "mark" the biliary system. For the purpose of the PTC the fasting patient receives premedication (Valium, atropine), a local anaesthetic (e.g. lignocaine), and antibiotic cover, and is placed in the supine position; the puncture is then made using the lateral transperitoneal approach. The lateral approach has the advantage that the whole mass of the liver acts as a protection against bile leakage. The biliary systen is punctured near the right hepatic duct just above the bifurcation, as this is commonly obstructed by tumour growth. In determining the site of the right hepatic duct, one uses the point of attachment of the diaphragm to the vertebrae as a reference point, aiming approximately 1½ to 2 vertebral bodies caudally. As a rule, the right hepatic duct is found at the level of the 12th thoracic vertebra, about 4 cm lateral to the midline. The highest intercostal space possible is chosen for the percutaneous approach, so that the Chiba needle can be advanced in a parallel plane to the large bile ducts in the liver, as this path is the most practical for the second puncture made for the purpose of drainage. In this way the necessity for two puncture sites can be avoided. Penetration of the phrenicocostal sinus is not accompanied by a higher complication rate as long as the anaesthetic is adequate and puncture is not performed during inspiration.

In a patient with a distance of 20 cm between table surface and sternum, the lateral puncture site is about 12 cm above the surface of the table top, while in the case of a smaller table top/sternum distance the site lies about 11 cm above the table surface (Fig. 20). It is recommended that the puncture is performed in a strictly horizontal plane, as this is the plane parallel to the path of the large intrahepatic bile ducts and allows greater accuracy. In addition, the danger of a biliovascular fistula is reduced as the vessels lie dorsal to the path of puncture.

If the needle deviates dorsally, the possibility of penetrating the liver capsule at the back or of puncturing the gallbladder arises. The puncture needle is advanced to its target point during apnoea in the midcycle of respiration. Unlike the method using a Teflon needle, during which a flow of bile indicates the position of the needle in an intrahepatic bile duct, with the Chiba needle it is necessary to inject contrast medium under slight pressure, owing to the narrow lumen. The distribution pattern of the extravasating contrast medium shows the position of the needle:

- If a pool of contrast medium forms that is only slowly absorbed, the end of the needle lies in liver parenchyma.
- If a portal vein has been punctured, the contrast medium rapidly flows towards the periphery; puncture of a hepatic vein results in a flow in a cranial direction to the left.
- Lymph vessels are seen as thin threat-like structures in the region of the hilus.
- The biliary system shows up as a band-like opacification that very rapidly spreads to the hilus and finally fills the remaining bile ducts in a retrograde fashion.

The number of attempts at puncture is not included in the complication rate as long as the capsule of the liver is not repeatedly punctured with each new attempt. *Okuda* et al. (1974), and *Ariyama* et al. (1978) make up to ten attempts at puncture.

Once it is certain that the end of the Chiba needle is lying in an intrahepatic bile duct, 10–30 ml contrast medium is injected to achieve good visualisation of the extrahepatic biliary system. For an optimal assessment of the intrahepatic and posthepatic bile ducts it is frequently necessary to turn the patient temporarily on his left side (for better filling of the left hepatic ducts) and to bring him into an erect position (to improve visualisation of the obstruction). As at this point there is very great danger of dislocation it is recommended to wait with the diagnostic part of the procedure until the drainage catheter has been inserted.

The second step consists of a second puncture of the contrast medium-filled biliary system with a Teflon needle catheter such as was used up to a few years ago for normal PTC. The second puncture is necessary as the Chiba needle does not allow passage of a guide wire into the biliary system to permit catheter exchange.

As soon as the puncture instrument has been introduced into the liver the introducing needle is removed. Then the Teflon catheter is slowly pulled back until there is a flow of bile. It may be necessary to make several attempts at puncture, and care must be taken not to let the catheter slip out of the liver whilst pulling it back, as during PTC, to avoid having to damage the liver capsule by a second stab. Once bile flows out of the catheter the guide wire is inserted in the bile duct and advanced to the obstruction or, whenever possible, across the stenosis into the duodenum (for internal drainage; Fig. 21).

The third step in this three-stage catheterisation procedure consists in exchanging the Teflon catheter over the guide wire by the conventional Seldinger technique for a 5-F or 7-F polyethylene catheter. It is helpful to dilate the puncture channel through the chest wall and liver capsule with a firmer, thicker Teflon catheter as dilator.

An attempt should always be made to push the drainage catheter through the stenosis or obstruction into the duodenum to allow internal drainage. The catheter used for this purpose has side-holes above as well as below the stenosis, to allow bile to flow out of the liver through the drain into the duodenum. Inadvertent drainage to the exterior of a well-functioning internal drainage system can be prevented by clamping the exterior part of the tubing so that all the bile formed in the liver drains physiologically into the duodenum.

If liver function is preserved or recovering, bile duct drainage generally results in a rapid drop or even a return to normal levels of the serum bilirubin within 1–2

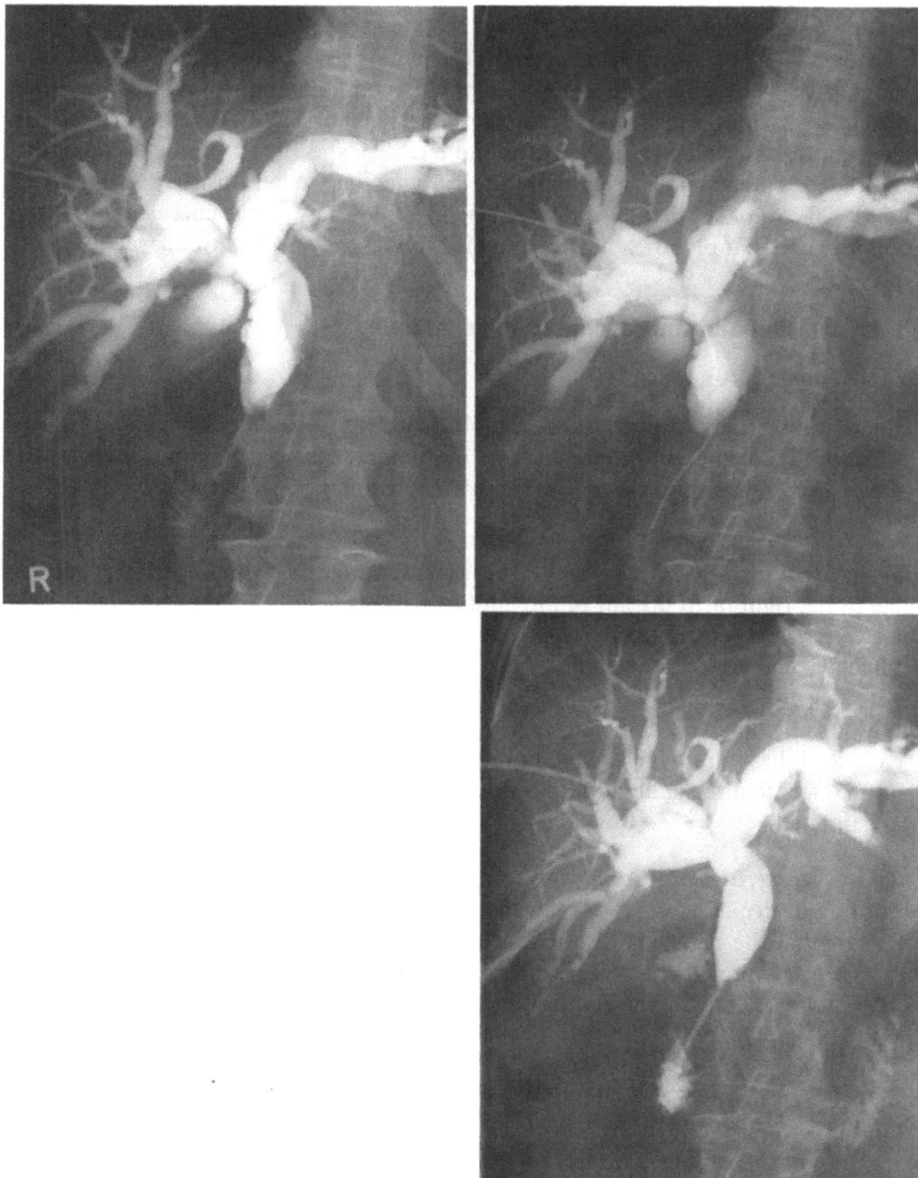

a b c

Fig. 21 a–c. A long stenotic segment due to metastases obstructing the common bile duct in a 72-year-old patient. Technical procedure of internal PTD. **a** Contrast-filled intra- and extrahepatic biliary channels with a high degree of stenosis in the distal common bile duct (PTC). **b** Insertion, through the puncture needle, of a guide wire, which is advanced through the stricture into the duodenum. **c** Internal drainage catheter lying with its tip in the duodenum: the side-holes are draining the obstructed biliary region. The puncture needle has been exchanged for the catheter by the Seldinger technique with the aid of the guide wire which remains in situ

weeks and an improvement in the general condition of the patient with relief of the frequently unbearable pruritis.

Management of the patients after PTD consists in an observation period of a minimum of 24 h to recognise any abdominal symptoms indicating sepsis, bilious peritonitis, or intra-abdominal or subcapsular haemorrhage. The drained bile is subjected to bacteriological investigation to enable a specific antibiotic treatment to be initiated if necessary. Twice daily the catheter has to be flushed several times with 10–20 cm^3 of sterile physiological NaCl solution to prevent encrustation – It is recommended that blood-chemistry and electrolytes are checked twice weekly.

5.3 Discussion and Improvement of Technique

5.3.1 Methods of Approach

Puncture of the liver for purposes of radiological demonstration of the bile duct system can be performed in different ways: by the anterior transperitoneal approach, by the lateral transperitoneal or posterior extraperitoneal approach, or transvenously.

Anterior Transperitoneal Approach. The puncture is carried out in the epigastric angle to the right or to the left of the midline (*Atkinson* et al. 1960; *Carter* and *Saypol* 1952; *Nurick* et al. 1953; *Remolar* et al. 1956; *Shaldon* et al. 1962), or in the medioclavicular line on the right (*Evans* 1973; *Felci* and *Felci* 1957; *Flemma* et al. 1963; *Isley* and *Schauble* 1962; *Kidd* 1950; *Peiper* et al. 1967; *Santos* et al. 1960). A few groups of Japanese clinicians, e.g. *Takada* et al. (1976) prefer this anterior approach for biliary drainage as they find the lateral approach more difficult. *Swart* et al. (1976) feel that the gallbladder, as described by *Peiper* et al. (1967), should not be overestimated.

Lateral Transperitoneal Approach. The puncture is carried out as described above. According to *Peiper* et al. (1967) the advantage of this method over the anterior approach is that the needle is inserted in the direction of the large bile ducts, so that these are easily punctured. According to *Swart* et al. (1976), the risk of biliovascular fistulas is lower, as the vessels lie dorsal to the large intra- and extrahepatic bile ducts (*Nettelblad* 1954).

We have tried both methods and can find no difference in the degree of difficulty between the two methods of puncture. As the lateral approach is more practical in that it offers a long intrahepatic channel, thus reducing the likelihood of a displacement of the catheter, we have decided in favour of the lateral approach. With the anterior approach we have observed that during PTC the needle catheter tends to slip out whilst the x-rays are being taken with the patient changing position. The only advantage that this method of approach offers is that the catheter sited in the parenchyma prevents any bleeding from the liver into the peritoneal cavity (*Swart* et al. 1976).

Posterior Extrahepatic Approach. This method exploits the fact that the dorsal attachment of the liver to the posterior thoracic wall is not covered by peritoneum. *Prioton* (1960) recommended this approach for liver biopsy and for PTC, as avoiding the peritoneum precludes any danger of bilious peritonitis. The probability that this technique will be successful is about 80%, and thus similar to that for the other methods.

The dorsal approach, however, is quite impractical for PTD and it is never used for this purpose.

Transvenous Transhepatic Approach. The transvenous transhepatic approach to cholangiography was introduced in 1967 by *Hanafee* and *Weiner* (1967) to avoid a percutaneous transhepatic puncture associated with the danger of biliary peritonitis and intraperitoneal bleeding. This method involves introduction of a special catheter needle system percutaneously into the internal jugular vein – preferably the right jugular vein – down through the superior vena cava, right atrium, and inferior vena cava into a hepatic vein. Under radiological control the catheter needle is manipulated across the vein wall and liver parenchyma to puncture an adjacent bile duct.

The success rate of this technique ranges from 65%–93% with dilatation, and between 10% and 69.5% without dilatation of the biliary system (*Günther* et al. 1980; *Hines* et al. 1972; *Kadell* and *Weiner* 1973; *Rösch* et al. 1975; *Tabrisky* et al. 1976; *Teisseive* et al. 1978; *Thelen* et al. 1977). The modification of using an arm vein as a method of approach, as suggested by *Hawkins* et al. (1976), does not offer any improvement of this method.

The complication rate of transvenous transhepatic cholangiography for the 495 cases published to date is quoted at 8.9% (mild complications 5.5%, serious complications, e.g. biliovenous fistulas, subcapsular hematomas of the liver, septicaemia 3.4%), with a mortality rate of 0.4% (as a result of septicaemia (*Günther* et al. 1980). If accuracy of procedure, morbidity and mortality of transvenous transhepatic cholangiography are compared with those of percutaneous transhepatic fine-needle cholangiography (without drainage) (Table 1), and the time and personnel involved

Table 1. Puncture accuracy, morbidity and mortality of transvenous cholangiography and percutaneous transhepatic fine-needle cholangiography. (From *Günther* et al. 1979)

	No. of cases	Accuracy of puncture		Morbidity	Mortality
		Obstruction	No obstruction		
Transvenous cholangiography	495	67%– 93%	10%–69.5%	8.9% (Mild complications 5.5%; severe complications 3.4%)	0.4%
Percutaneous transhepatic fine-needle cholangiography	2330	90%–100%	25%–89%	13.2% (Mild complications 10.1% [a]; severe complications 3.1%)	0.086%

[a] The higher percentage of mild complications with percutaneous transhepatic fine-needle cholangiography can be explained by the large number of pain reactions reported by certain authors (*Ariyama* et al. 1978; *Benjamin* et al. 1978; *Dammermann* et al. 1978)

and the need for greater angiographic experience and manual dexterity for the first method are also taken into account, it appears that transvenous cholangiography is not at all useful.

The value of this method is limited to the venography of hepatic and portal veins. Attempted transvenous transhepatic biliary drainage as a sequel to transvenous cholangiography has never been described; it seems it would be quite impractical.

5.3.2 Catheterisation Techniques

The most popular method is three-stage catheterisation, consisting of identification of the biliary system by means of the ultrathin Chiba needle, a second puncture of the contrast-filled biliary system with a Teflon needle catheter to insert a guide wire of normal thickness, and replacement of the Teflon needle catheter by a drainage catheter (*Hoevels* et al. 1978; *Ring* et al. 1978; *Takada* et al. 1976).

Some groups of clinicians consider a second puncture of the liver too hazardous, and use quite a long Teflon needle catheter (27 cm in length; ID/OD 1.0/1.6 mm) from the outset, advancing it into the biliary system and in some cases exchanging it for a thicker polyethylene catheter (ID/OD 1.4/2.2 mm) (*Burcharth* and *Nielbo* 1976; *Tylén* et al. 1977).

Günther et al. (1979) employed a fine needle (OD 0.5 mm; length 10 or 14 cm) to puncture the bile ducts, and also an ultrathin guide wire (OD 0.2 mm). Following the principle of step-by-step dilatation, they use a coaxial technique to exchange catheter needles and guide wires of increasing diameter up to a guide wire diameter of 1.0 mm. Over this they then insert a 5-F polyethylene drainage catheter.

In our opinion, three-stage catheterisation with a Chiba needle also has its drawbacks:

1. Despite a biliary system already filled with contrast medium and the radiological screening, the second puncture can turn out to be difficult, particularly if there are no facilities for screening in two planes.

2. In contrast to the thick Teflon needle catheter, during puncture with the Chiba needle the correct position cannot be confirmed by an outflow of bile. Instead, it is necessary to inject contrast medium. If the needle tip lies in the liver parenchyma pools of contrast medium form, thus rendering diagnosis more difficult. With the needle in the correct position there is also a further rise in pressure in the congested biliary system, caused by the injection of contrast medium; this is associated with a higher incidence of bacteraemia or sepsis.

According to *Irish* and *Meany* (1980) the success rates of PTC in the presence of a dilated biliary system lie around 94.2% with the Chiba needle and around 94.1% with the Teflon catheter needle, which is roughly twice as thick, i.e., are of the same order. Our results agree with these figures: in 243 PTCs performed, success rates of 94% with the Chiba needle and 92.4% with the needle catheter were obtained.

The number of attempts at puncture greatly influences the success rate. Figures obtained from a large American collective (*Bear* 1977) showed that groups of clinicians making a maximum of six attempts at puncture had a significantly lower success rate than those making six or more attempts. The number of attempts at puncture is not related to the complication rate, however, as long as care is taken

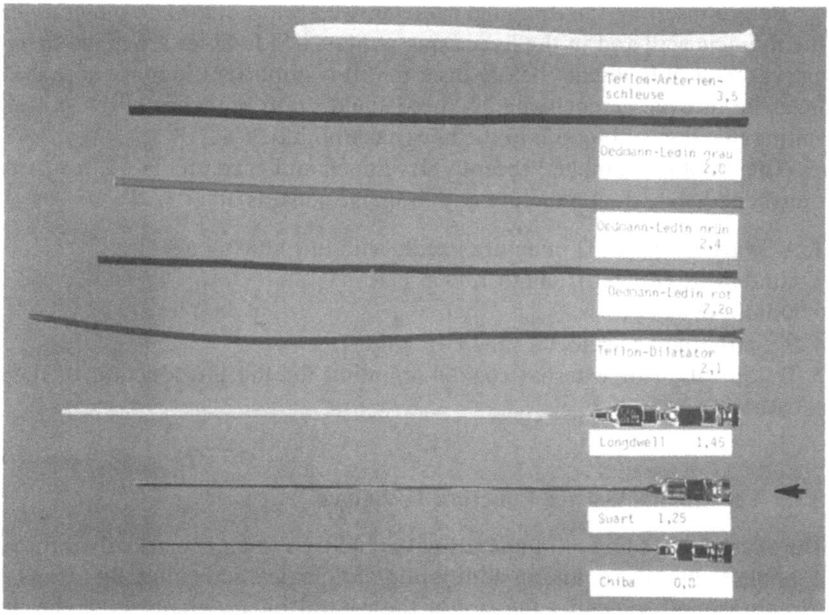

Fig. 22. Comparison of sizes of puncture needles, dilators, drainage catheters and arterial locks. The Swart PTD puncture needle is between the Chiba needle and the LONGWELL-Teflon needle catheter in external diameter

during repeated attempts to use the same site of entry on the surface of the liver, as already mentioned.

The total complication rate for PTC (including only serious complications such as bile leakage, intraperitoneal bleeding, death of the patient) according to collective figures published by *Harbin* et al. (1980) is about 1.5% for the Chiba needle and 5.5% for the Teflon needle catheter. The significant difference in complication rates may apply to pure PTC, but not to cases with subsequent decompression drainage.

Bearing in mind that it was essential (1) not to reduce the accuracy and (2) not to increase the complication rate, Swart and Köster developed a new needle (Fig. 22). This needle has a thin wall and a special tip rather like the Chiba needle. The outer diameter of 1.25 mm makes it thicker than the Chiba needle (OD 0.8 mm) but thinner than the Teflon needle catheter normally used (OD 1.45 mm or 1.6 mm).

The Swart needle offers the following advantages:

1. Bile can easily be aspirated, enabling one to judge whether the needle lies in position in the biliary system without an injection of contrast medium;
2. Before the biliary system is filled with contrast medium bile can be drained off, thus preventing bacteraemia or septicaemia that might be caused by injecting under pressure into a congested biliary system;
3. It is possible to avoid a second puncture and to introduce a PE 160 guide wire into the biliary system through the puncture needle; the needle can then be exchanged over the guide wire for a 7-F or larger dilator or drainage catheter (or 5-F or larger for children).

Before inserting the drainage catheter, we always dilate the puncture channel in the thoracic wall and in the liver using a dilator. Side-holes are made in each drainage catheter individually before insertion. It is important to make sure that no side-holes lie in liver parenchyma, as these could drain branches of the portal vein, resulting in a flow of blood into the bile (haemobilia).

The set of instruments[2] recently developed and currently in use for percutaneous transhepatic bile duct puncture and drainage consists of:

1. A Swart special PTD puncture needle with introducing needle
2. Guide wire (PE 160), length 1.00 m
3. Dilator (6–7 F)
4. Pig-tail drainage catheter (5/7 F or larger)
5. Teflon tube (for external coaxial splinting for the introduction of the drainage catheter)

5.3.3 Ultrasound-Assisted Puncture Technique

The accuracy obtained in puncturing the biliary system is markedly improved if it is possible to use ultrasound in addition to radiological screening. By means of epigastric ultrasound screening the site of the central biliary channels or the hepatic bifurcation can be located and marked on the skin. This marking serves as a reliable target for the transperitoneal puncture performed by a lateral approach and under radiological screening. If the first attempt at puncture does not result in successful entry of a biliary duct, further ultrasound examination over the epigastric region allows identification of the topographical relation between the point of the puncture needle and the dilated bile ducts in a longitudinal and transverse plane, which permits a well-aimed puncture of an adjacent bile duct. Since adopting this technique we have only needed to make two to three attempts at puncture.

In our opinion, lateral puncture guided exclusively by ultrasound using a puncturing transducer is currently not very practical, as a puncturing procedure followed by removal of the transducer from the indwelling puncture needle is too awkward and time consuming compared with the fluoroscopic (DL)-guided method. There is also an increased risk of lacerating the liver capsule, and the subsequent insertion of a guide wire and exchange of the puncture needle for the drainage catheter cannot be screened adequately with ultrasound alone.

5.4 Types of Drainage

There are two types of percutaneous transhepatic biliary drainage depending on the positioning of the drainage catheters.

---

2 Available from Messrs. Heinrich C. Ulrich, Workshops for Medical Mechanics, 7900 Ulm, West Germany (Tel. 07 31/6 00 01)

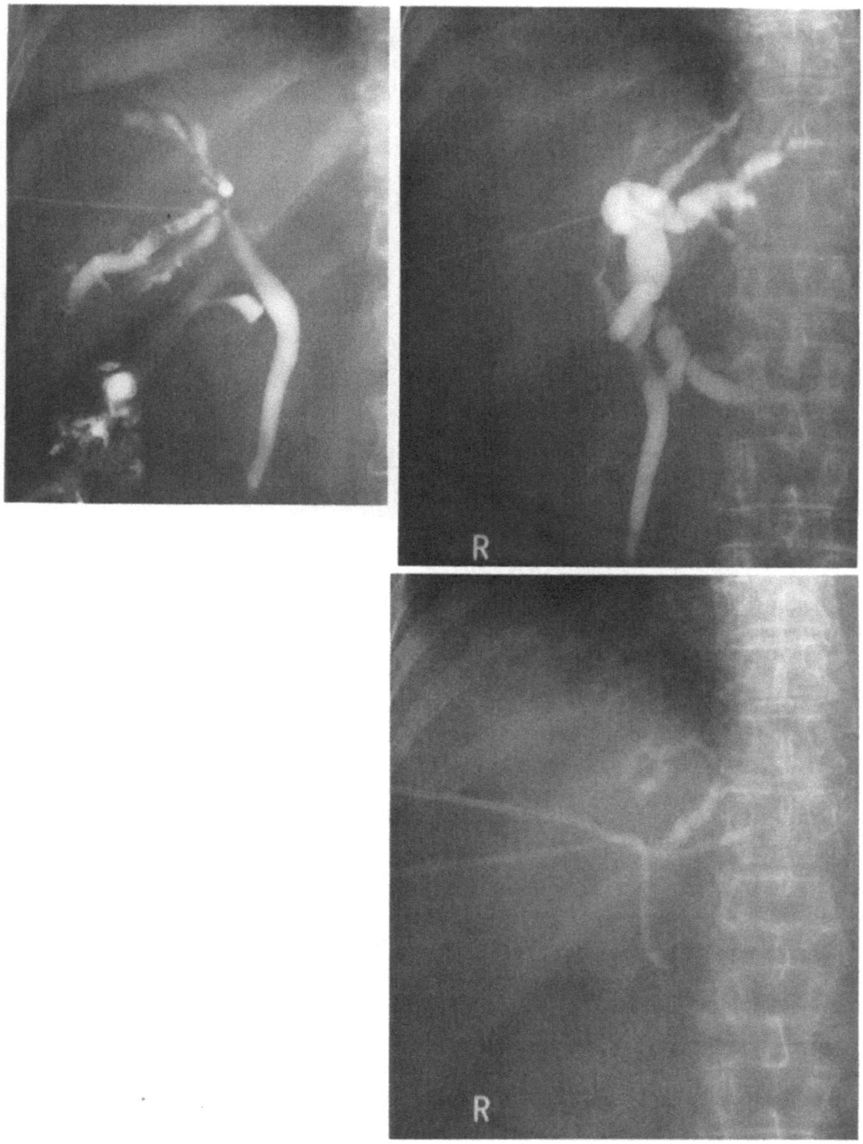

a b c

Fig. 23 a–c. Adenocarcinoma of the liver, metastases in the hilar region of the liver and obstruction of the hepatic bifurcation in a 71-year-old female patient. **a** PTC of the right hepatic bile duct reveals a tight stenosis of the right hepatic duct in the region of the confluence. **b** PTC of the left hepatic bile duct reveals a long, severely stenotic segment in the left hepatic duct in the region of the confluence. **c** External PTD with two catheters was inserted, one catheter being in the region of the right hepatic duct, the other in the region of the left hepatic duct

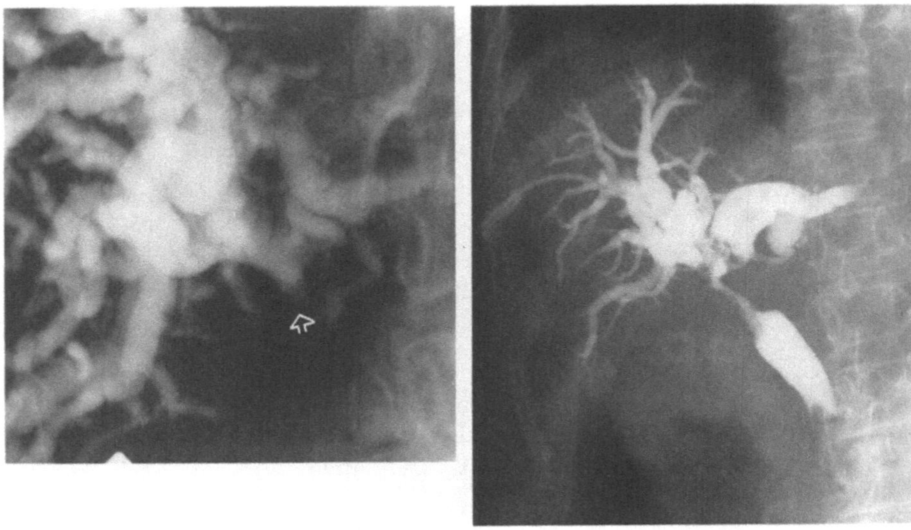

a b

Fig. 24 a, b. Extensive carcinoma of the gallbladder and metastases in the hilar lymph nodes in an 82-year-old female patient. **a** Highly localised, complete occlusion of the common hepatic bile duct just distal to the hepatic bifurcation. **b** Decompression by means of PTD has caused the completely obstructed common hepatic bile duct to open up, allowing visualisation of a long, tightly stenotic segment in the proximal part of the common hepatic bile duct

5.4.1 Internal

In internal PTD (see Fig. 21) the tip of the catheter is in the duodenum. The catheter is positioned in such a way that there are side-holes both above and below the obstruction or stricture; the side-holes in the catheter are sited specifically according to the findings of the PTC carried out beforehand. The correct positioning of the catheter is indicated by easy aspiration of bile and good opacification of the biliary system and duodenum after an injection of contrast medium.

As a rule, the internal drain is initially also drained to the outside for a few days, producing a bile flow of about 600–800 cm^3/day. A reduction of bile flow after a few days (to about 100–200 cm^3/day) implies that the internal drainage is functioning well. The external part of the catheter can then be closed, but remains accessible for catheter changes and washouts. Whatever the cause of the biliary obstruction, internal drainage should always be attempted, as this prevents the patient losing his bile. After PTC it frequently appears that the obstruction is complete, but this can be overcome by the guide wire, enabling internal drainage.

5.4.2 External

For the purpose of external drainage, the catheter is advanced as far as possible to the site of obstruction in the hepatic bile duct and drained to the exterior. If the obstruction lies in the perihilar region of the liver, with congestion of several isolated parts of the intrahepatic biliary system, attempts should be made to drain the congested biliary ducts selectively (Fig. 23).

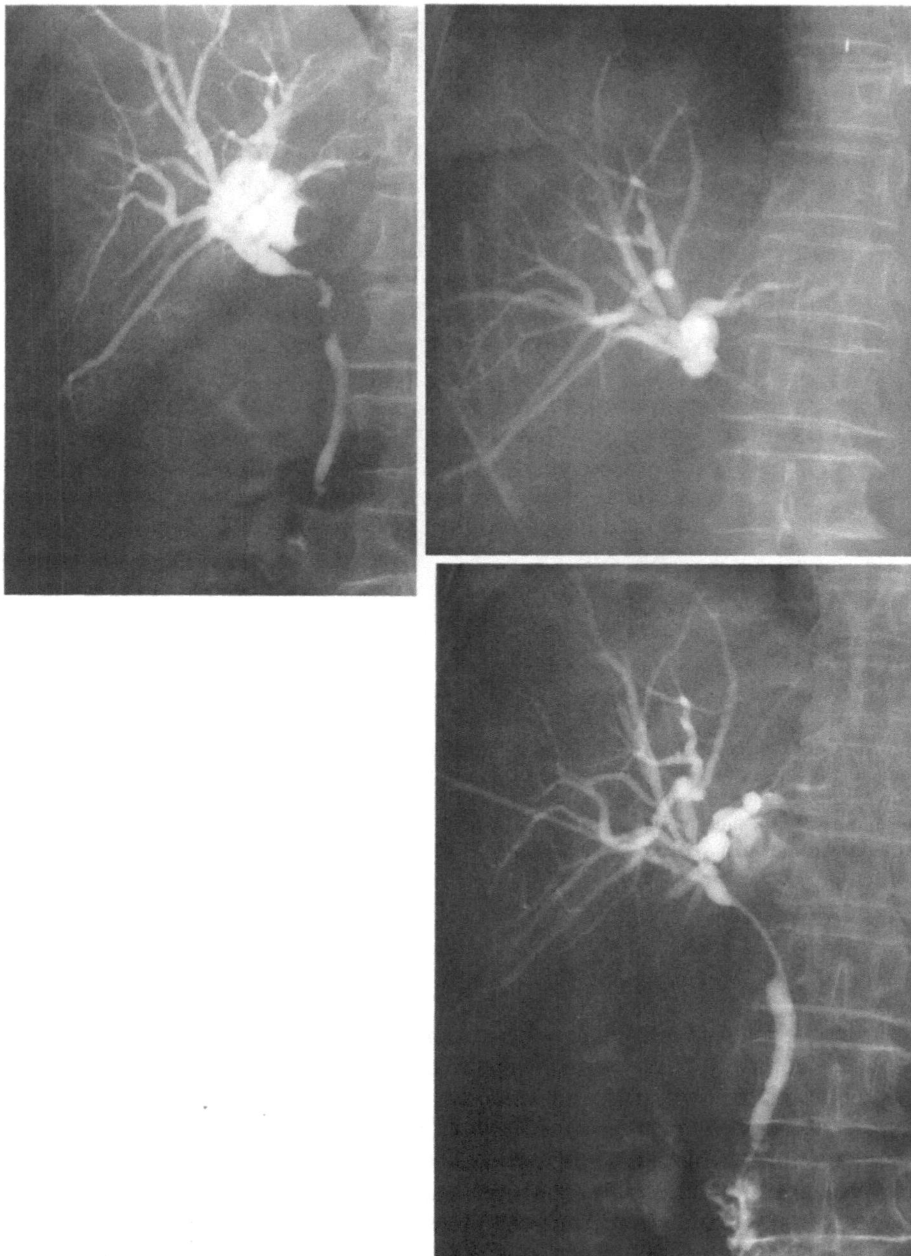

a b c

Fig. 25 a–c. Metastasising inoperable gallbladder carcinoma in a 73-year-old female patient. **a** PTC reveals several tight strictures of the common hepatic bile duct in series. **b** External PTD is shown in situ, with the catheter tip lying in front of the uppermost malignant stricture. **c** For conversion of external to internal drainage the catheter is advanced through the stenotic region into the duodenum. There are side-holes above as well as below the stenotic region

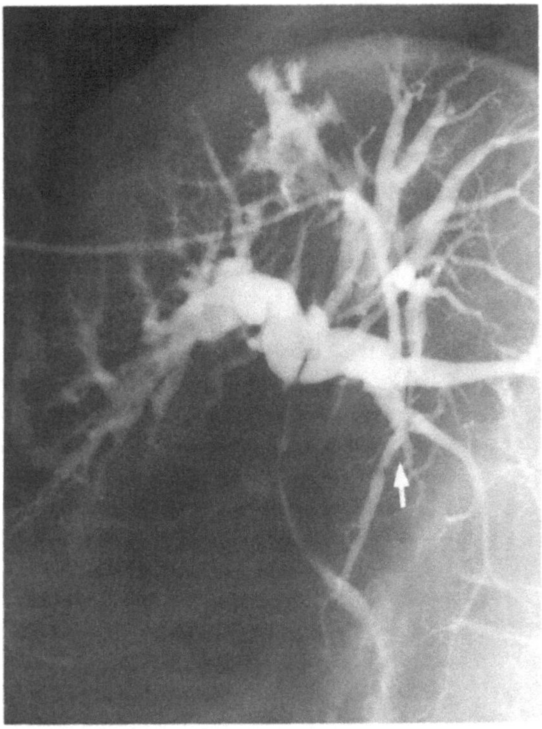

Fig. 26. Bile duct carcinoma in a 64-year-old female patient. A long, markedly stenotic segment in the common hepatic bile duct begins in the region of the confluence. The a.p. view showed the catheter tip lying centrally in front of the stenosis and indicated that internal drainage is possible; in fact, however, this proved to be impossible. The lateral view shows that the catheter viewed in a second plane is lying with its tip not in a central position but in the periphery

5.4.3 Conversion of External to Internal

After decongestion of the biliary system, some extremely narrow strictures that appeared as complete obstructions in the PTC may become patent again (Fig. 24), making it possible to exchange the external catheter for an internal drainage catheter over an indwelling guide wire, and thus converting the external drainage to an internal drainage. This can be done provided the external drainage catheter is suitably positioned: the tip should lie in a central branch of the liver (Fig. 25). In a few isolated cases this can only be assessed by screening in a second plane, as the illusion of a centrally positioned catheter may be produced by screening in just one plane (Fig. 26).

6 Discussion of the Method

6.1 Typical Problems with PTD

6.1.1 Difficulties in Introduction of the Catheter

Usually the drainage catheter can be introduced into the liver and the biliary system with ease using the Seldinger technique of passing it over the guide wire. In one series of cases we observed kinking of the catheter and guide wire against the liver, or later after the tip of the catheter had been advanced into the biliary system, which made it very difficult to push the catheter up to the obstruction (Fig. 27). This is due partly to the choice of catheter material: polyethylene catheters are very pliable and tend to kink easily during introduction into the liver. On the other hand, catheter kinking always occurs during introduction into the biliary system when vigorous manipulation in the thoracic wall causes air to penetrate between liver and thoracic wall, resulting in a pneumoperitoneum. The same problem is encountered when the distance between liver and thoracic wall is increased by ascites. Difficulties are also more frequently encountered with cirrhotic or metastatic livers. The combination of a rigid system at the surface (in this case between thoracic wall and liver surface) and a softer system deeper down (in this case liver parenchyma) poses problems already familiar in transfemoral angiography, where they have been solved by the use of arterial locks. These have also been used for our purposes; the Teflon tubes of the arterial locks are introduced into the liver over the polyethylene catheter with the guide wire already in place in the liver parenchyma by means of the same technique as in angiography, and the catheter is subsequently advanced over the same guide wire and through the locks (Fig. 28).

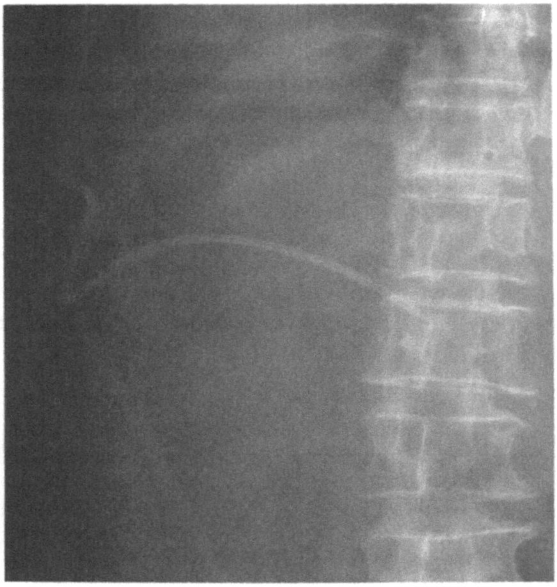

Fig. 27. Metastasising inoperable gallbladder carcinoma in a 73-year-old female patient. A curved kink is seen in the drainage catheter between chest wall and liver

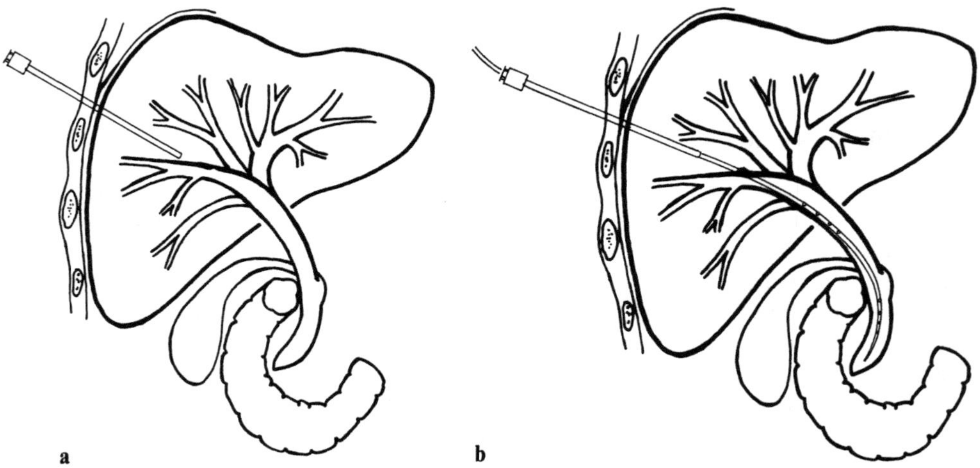

a b

Fig. 28a, b. Use of the arterial locks in PTD: **a** Teflon lock lying in the chest wall and liver; **b** PTD catheter being inserted through the Teflon lock into the biliary system

We now use the Teflon tubes of the Swart arterial locks in about 95% of PTDs and no longer experience difficulties with the introduction of the drainage catheters. As soon as the drainage catheter is in the biliary system and bile is flowing freely the Teflon tube is completely withdrawn. We have not observed any increased risk of biliary extravasation or bleeding during use of the Teflon tubes, despite their frequent use and larger outer diameter (3.5 mm).

Another point in favour of using locks is that catheters of different diameters can be exchanged as often as required without an increased risk of biliary extravasation, as there is no new puncture of the liver or marked dilatation of the puncture canal.

Pereiras et al. (1977) and *Takada* et al. (1976) use similar methods, whilst *Hoevels* et al. (1978) solve the problem by using a rigid guide wire, 80 cm in length and 0.9 mm in diameter, with a long flexible segment for the tip, which is available in two lengths, 8 cm or 12 cm. In our opinion, it seems probable that the latter would cause considerable trauma to the liver and is rather impractical.

6.1.2 Catheter Displacement

A frequent problem of PTD, but one which usually has no clinical sequelae, is posed by the catheter slipping out of the liver during sneezing, coughing, or body movement, despite the lateral approach. The catheter ends up in the liver parenchyma or between thoracic wall and diaphragm.

Catheter displacement always occurs when drainage is external and a high obstruction only allows a short intrahepatic portion of catheter. We therefore pushed the catheter as far in as possible, irrespective of the site of the obstruction, either as far as the obstruction in the hepatic bile duct or a long way into the left bile duct or even cranially into a larger branch (Fig. 29). We now use a so-called pig-tail catheter in every case of external drainage; the curved end of the pig-tail catheter braces against the walls of the bile duct thus anchoring the catheter (Fig. 30).

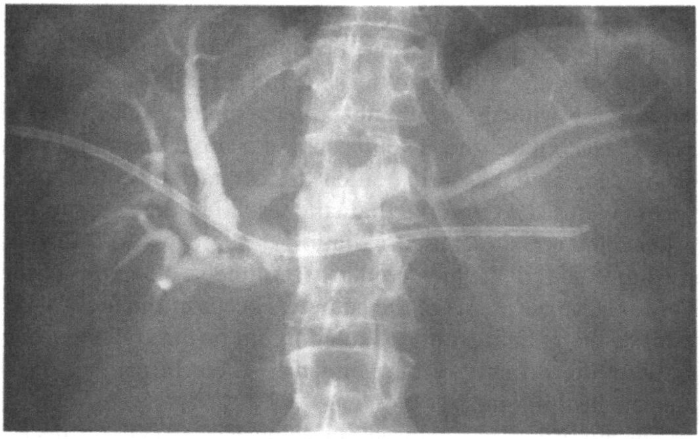

Fig. 29. Gallbladder carcinoma and central metastases in a 66-year-old patient: the free end of the external drainage catheter has been advanced far into the region of the left hepatic duct for better stabilisation

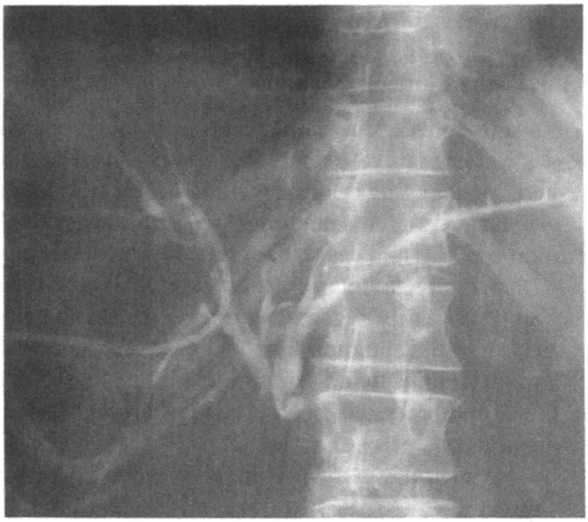

Fig. 30. Obstruction of the common bile duct due to metastases from an ovarian carcinoma in a 57-year-old female patient. External PTD was instituted, the drainage catheter being anchored with a pig-tail-like end in the periphery of the right hepatic duct region

An alternative way of securing the drainage catheter more effectively in the biliary system is the use of balloon catheters. When an arterial lock is used, the introduction of such balloon catheters should not present any problems, contrary to the opinion of *Hansson* et al. (1979). Some difficulties are still encountered in making such balloon catheters with a sufficiently large internal lumen and an individual arrangement of side-holes distal to the baloon. The best way, of course, of preventing dislodgement of the drainage catheter is the method of internal drainage, i.e., advancing the catheter through a bile duct stricture right into the duodenum.

Fixing the drainage catheters to the skin to prevent displacement is only important in very active, agitated or uncooperative patients. We used to put a lot of effort into stitching the catheter to the skin and carefully choosing the suture material suitable for use with the synthetic catheter material (*Köster* et al. 1979), but now we merely attach the catheter to the skin in a curved fashion by means of adhesive plaster and, for added security, stitch the catheter onto the strips of plaster in several places. We used to observe that stitches fixing the catheter to skin directly adjacent to the puncture site caused irritation of the chest wall through constant tension of the suture material, which regularly resulted in infections of the thoracic wall.

Most displacements of the catheters occur in the first 24–48 hours after PTD as a result of the patient sitting or standing up or through vigorous respiratory efforts. It is, therefore, strongly recommended to keep the patient on bedrest for about 48 h after the institution of PTD.

The time that has elapsed since the PTC/PTD is a decisive factor for the correction of a catheter displacement. Early dislocations demand a repeat PTC with subsequent drainage. In the case of dislodgement of the drainage catheter after a longer period of time, it is generally possible to insert a new guide wire catheter system, and to re-use the previous puncture channel which will be lined with connective tissue.

6.1.3 Faulty Catheter Positions

If the side-holes of the catheter lie in liver parenchyma, and are draining a larger vessel, rather marked haemobilia occurs. This can be corrected by repositioning the catheter or changing it for one with a different number of side-holes.

Mild haemobilia, sometimes persisting for several hours, occurs in a large proportion of PTDs and ceases spontaneously without any problems.

Other faulty catheter positions are characterised by an incorrect path of puncture and are easily recognised during a radiological check: entry of the drainage catheter into the common bile duct or cystic duct, without or after traversing the liver and exciting at the lower surface of the liver (Fig. 31). Provided no side-holes lie in the abdominal cavity, complications are unlikely, particularly as these cases subsequently undergo operation.

In our method, involving the choice of a high puncture site and a steep passage of the catheter towards the hilus of the liver, penetration of the phrenical costal angle is not considered faulty or in need of correction. We have never observed complications such as pneumothorax or bilious pleural effusion.

6.1.4 Catheter Obstruction

Cell debris, encrustation, formation of blood and bile clots, or ingrowth of tumour can cause obstruction of the catheter. This has clinical implications, such as cessation of bile flow out of the catheter, a renewed rise in bilirubin levels, bile leakage between the catheter and the opening of the drainage canal along the thoracic wall, or the occurrence of infection.

Injection of a contrast medium into the catheter confirms the diagnosis. Treatment consists, first of all, in attempting to clear the catheter by forced washouts, or to recanalise the catheter by using a guide wire and exchanging the catheter for a

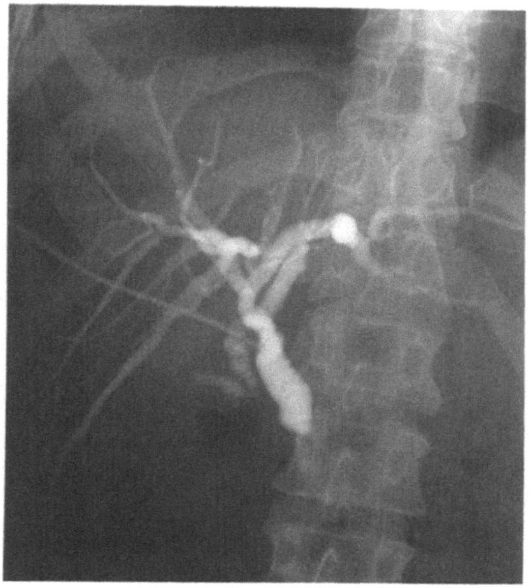

Fig. 31. Carcinoma of the head of the pancreas 8 mm in diameter in a 50-year-old female patient. Faulty positioning of the external PTD: the catheter enters the common bile duct subhepatically from the dorsal aspect after traversing the liver and exiting at the lower surface of the liver

new one by the Seldinger technique. If the recanalisation of the catheter is unsuccessful an attempt at exchanging the obstructed catheter for a new one by means of coaxial external splinting is recommended. The Teflon tube (described above) is advanced over the indwelling drainage catheter into the biliary system (Fig. 28); the obstructed catheter can then be removed and a new catheter (with a guide wire for easier introduction) inserted. The Teflon tube is afterwards retracted. If the newly inserted catheter results in free drainage of the biliary system complications are not likely to result from the use of a thicker Teflon tube.

6.1.5 Persistence of Jaundice Despite Drainage

Persisting hyperbilirubinaemia or rising serum bilirubin despite an indwelling drainage catheter may be attributable to one of the following situations:

1. Unsatisfactory bile drainage through the catheter because it has either too small an internal diameter or an insufficient number of side-holes. We use the 7-F polyethylen catheter (OD/ID 2.2 mm/1.4 mm) with side-holes that guarantee an adequate flow of bile according to trials conducted by *Hansson* et al. (1979), i.e. 8 ml/min with a pressure of 10 cmH_2O or 5.5 ml/min with a pressure of 5 cmH_2O.

2. Obstruction of the catheter (or of its side-holes). In this case the catheter has to be flushed through, possibly recanalised, preferably exchanged for a new one.

3. Failure of congested parts of the biliary system to drain. In this case it is necessary to try and visualise the sites of bile duct obstruction and to drain these regions separately. Our experience shows that hyperbilirubinaemia persists if only partial decongestion of the biliary system is achieved (Fig. 32). This is in contrast to

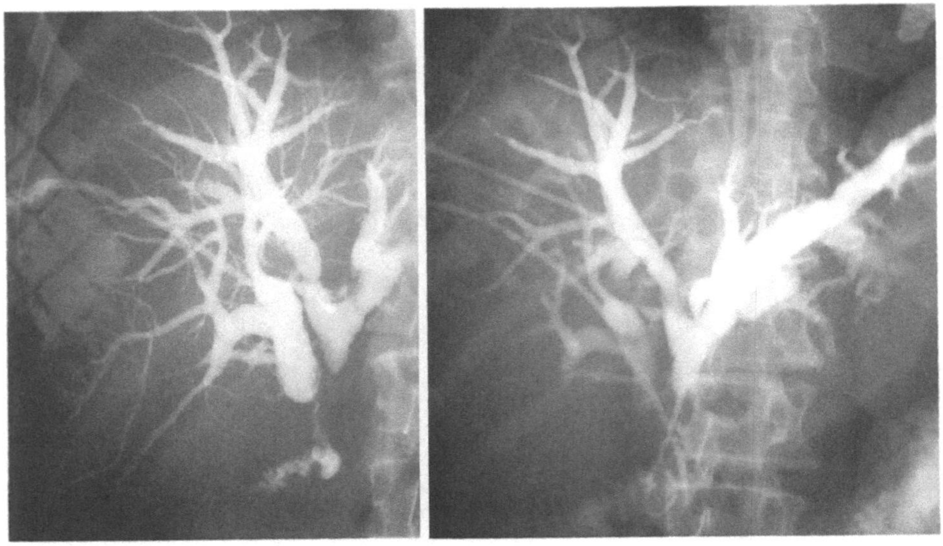

a b

Fig. 32 a, b. Recurrence of a biliary duct carcinoma after previous hepaticojejunostomy in a 57-year-old patient. **a** External drainage of the right hepatic duct region. Opacification of the region drained by the left hepatic duct which is also, but separately, obstructed. **b** Adequate relief of the obstruction was achieved only after two simultaneous internal drainage systems had been constructed

the views of *Cahow* (1979), who merely considers it necessary to relieve the obstruction of only one lobe of the liver (in this case surgically). *Roux* and *Larimore* demonstrated in 1920 that obstruction of the biliary system of one lobe of the liver results in hypertrophy of the contralateral liver lobe, which takes over the full function of the liver whilst the obstructed lobe atrophies. This observation is contrary to our own experience.

4. Progressive liver damage caused by tumour growth or irreversibly damaged liver parenchyma. Obstruction persisting for any length of time causes destruction of intralobular bile ducts, which is irreversible and provides an explanation for the persistence of hyperbilirubinaemia despite drainage.

6.2 Complications of PTD

Serious complications of PTD cannot be separated from those of PTC: infections with abscess formation, bile leakage, intraperitoneal bleeding and death. The total incidence of serious complications after PTD is quoted at 2.5% (*Hoevels* et al. 1978) to 5% (*Ferruci* et al. 1980); and after PTC (irrespective of subsequent PTD), in statistics collected by *Harbin* et al. (1980), at 1.5% with the Chiba needle and 5.5% with the Teflon needle catheter. Considering the course of disease for patients without PTD and the high mortality associated with attempted surgery, this very high complication rate for a diagnostic/therapeutic procedure seems quite tolerable and will most certainly be lowered as more experience is gained with PTD.

Harbin et al. (1980) reported three deaths amongst 2000 PTCs. Bile leakage occurred in 1%/3.5% and intraperitoneal bleeding in 0.3%/1.8% (Chiba-needle/needle catheter). These complications cause clinical symptoms in only a small proportion of patients, but then call for an emergency operation. In our opinion, both types of complication are reduced by the subsequent drainage procedure.

The main complication of PTD is generalised infection with rigors and fever accompanied by a drop in blood pressure, positive blood cultures or serious impairment of the patient's general condition. In patients with obstructive jaundice, the rate of infection of the bile ducts is 71%–90% in the presence to calculi, 25%–36% in the presence of tumours (*Keighley* 1977). During PTC with subsequent PTD there is frequently an influx of infected bile into the bloodstream through the direct connection between bile ducts and liver sinusoids. To avoid sepsis, PTC and PTD are performed under prophylactic antibiotic therapy. The antibiotics of choice are Gentamicin and Ampicillin, as there is a preponderance of *Escherichia coli, Klebsiella aerogenes* and *Streptococcus faecalis* in the infected bile. It is necessary to differentiate a sepsis-like shock within the first few hours after PTC/PTD, actual sepsis, and endotoxic shock that is not affected by prophylactic antibiotics but is readily managed with antipyretics and vasoactive drugs (if necessary, Dolantin).

Intrahepatic vascular trauma, as seen with liver biopsy and PTC (*Bear* 1977; *Göthlin* and *Transberg* 1973; *Hellekant* 1976; *Okuda* et al. 1978) might be frequently expected, but is only rarely reported: whereas in a group of 27 patients in whom PTD was performed *Luska* et al. (1981) did not observe a single case of intrahepatic bleeding or similar trauma in the 13 patients examined by CT after the procedure, *Tylen* et al. (1977) reported 10 cases of intrahepatic vascular trauma (4 with extravasation of contrast medium, 6 with arterial-portal shunts) in 65 patients subjected to arteriography after PTD. *Hoevels* et al. (1980a) had 27 cases (14 aneurysms, 7 haematomas, 7 arterio-portal fistulas) amongst 83 patients in whom post-PTD arteriography was performed.

These vascular complications usually do not cause any symptoms and heal spontaneously; in the remaining cases the treatment of choice consists of blood transfusions and, in a very few cases, intrahepatic embolisation.

It is surprisingly rare for tumour cells to spread along the drainage tract; only three cases have been reported to date in the world literature. *Hoevels* et al. (1978) and *Kim* et al. (1982) have each described a case of implantation metastasis in the skin around the puncture site 3 weeks and 5 months, respectively, after removal of the drainage catheter after operative construction of a biliodigestive anastomosis for management of carcinoma of the head of the pancreas. In a case report by *Olega* et al. (1980) implantation metastasis occurred 16 months after biliary drainage in a case of bile duct carcinoma.

7 Our Own Results

Between 1965 and the present day, 285 percutaneous transhepatic punctures have been performed in our institute, 103 of these with the Teflon needle catheter previously in use, 110 with a Chiba needle, and 72 with our own Swart needle. Of these

Table 2. Percutaneous transhepatic drainage ($n = 120$)

Successful:	116 Internal drainage 22 External drainage 94 Conversion of external to internal drainages 6	97.0%
Unsuccessful:	4	3.0%
Total number of patients: 106		
Number of patients with successful PTD: 102		

punctures, 225 have been successful. Jaundice was caused by malignant tumours in 214 cases and by calculi in 46 cases; other causes were found in only 25 cases.

Since November 1977 we have carried out 120 PTD procedures following PTC in 106 patients (45 drainages were for other hospitals); in four additional patients attempts at PTD were unsuccessful (Table 2). Although in one of these unsuccessful cases it was possible to introduce the drainage catheter into the hepatic bile duct right up to the obstruction (carcinoma of the pancreas), it was only possible to achieve aspiration of sticky black bile. Despite repeated alterations in the position of the catheter and extensive flushing, a free flow of bile was never obtained. The drainage procedure was therefore interrupted, and the patient underwent immediate operation. Massive bile thrombi were found intraoperatively in the biliary ducts and were washed out with great difficulty.

In the second unsuccessful case, haemorrhage occurred from the puncture channel during the percutaneous transhepatic bile duct puncture, requiring immediate operative intervention. It turned out that the cause of the bleeding was not poor puncture technique, but previously unrecognised severe portal hypertension, which also caused great surgical difficulties during intraoperative liver biopsies.

In the third unsuccessful case, the PTC showed only a slightly dilated intrahepatic biliary system in the presence of grossly dilated extrahepatic bile ducts, with transverse obliteration of the common bile duct and perforation into the abdominal cavity of a gallbladder filled with calculi. A larger bile duct suitable for insertion of a drainage catheter could not be found. The patient unfortunately died, despite a laparotomy immediately afterwards, as severe bilious peritonitis had already supervened.

In the case of the fourth patient in whom PTD was unsuccessful, extremely severe upper abdominal symptoms occurred during manipulation with the drainage catheter, so we discontinued the PTD procedure and arranged for immediate operation (in this case choledochojejunostomy).

The patient collective consisted of 64 women, 41 men, and 1 child. The youngest patient was 2 years old, the oldest 99 years of age. A definite preponderance of older people can be seen in the age distribution (Table 3).

All patients exhibited bile duct obstruction, with differing degrees of bile duct dilatation. Tumour was the cause of obstruction in 91 cases (=86%), mainly carcinomas of the head of the pancreas or bile duct carcinomas; in 15 cases (= 14%) the cause was benign (Table 4). In 15 patients anastomosing operations had already been performed because of a malignancy before PTD.

Table 3. Age distribution of patients

Age (years)	*n*	%
0– 9	1	1.0
10–19	–	–
20–29	–	–
30–39	2	2.0
40–49	5	4.5
50–59	17	16.0
60–69	24	22.5
70–79	42	40.0
80–89	14	13.0
90–99	1	1.0
	106	100.0

Table 4. Causes of biliary obstruction ($n = 106$)

Benign	
Calculus	6
Papillary stenosis	2
Secondary cholangitis	4
Anastomotic stricture	1
Common bile duct lesion	1
Pancreatic pseudocyst	1
	15 (14%)
Malignant	
Carcinoma of the head of pancreas	34
Bile duct carcinoma	19
Gallbladder carcinoma	19
Metastases	13
Liver cell carcinoma	4
Papillary carcinoma	2
	91 (86%)

Of the 116 successful PTDs, 22 (19%) were primarily constructed for internal drainage and 94 (81%) for external drainage (Table 2). O fthe external drainages, 6 were later converted to internal drainage. External drainage was used both in patients with a complete obliteration of the hepatic bile duct and in patients with multiple or tight stenoses in whom internal drainage failed.

PTD was performed twice in each of six patients and three times in another patient. Five patients with malignant obstruction at the confluence of the bile duct each had two simultaneous external drains in the two congested branches of the hepatic system, and one patient had two simultaneous internal drains. The drains remained in place for between 1 day and 3 years 4 months (Table 5), about 20% of cases falling into each of the groups with duration of drainage up to 1 week, 2 weeks, 1 month, and 2 months.

Table 5. Duration of PTD ($n = 102$)

Duration (days)	*n*	%
Up to 7	21	20.5
7– 14	17	16.5
14– 30	20	19.5
30– 60	25	24.5
60–180	12	12.0
180–365	4	4.0
Over 365	3	3.0

Table 6. Fall in serum bilirubin ($n = 102$)

Fall in bilirubin (mg %)	*n*	%
0– 5	31	30.25
5–10	32	31.25
10–20	33	32.5
Over 20	6	6.0

Subjective improvement of symptoms (pruritus, loss of appetite, poor general condition) was reported by 90% of the patients. In the patients without symptomatic improvement, the indications for PTD had obviously been recognised too late (they died within 10 days of PTD) or the operation was carried out too close to PTD.

With external drainage there was generally a daily biliary flow of between 300 and 800 ml (max. 1500 ml). The initial bilirubin values as an indication of the degree of jaundice were over 10 mg% in 46 patients (25 of whom had values over 20mg%). During drainage a fall in bilirubin levels by 5–10 mg% was achieved in 32 patients (31.25%) of 10–20 mg% in 33 patients (32.5%), and more than 20 mg% in six patients (6%) (Table 6). As a rule, the bilirubin levels fall fastest in the first 2 weeks. In the cases that did not respond well to drainage malignant growth was generally too far advanced, or secondary liver cell damage was irreversible, or surgery followed PTD so closely that there was too little time for a fall in bilirubin levels.

Of the 106 patients, 44 underwent surgery after PTD: 10 for a benign lesion and 34 for malignancy. One patient with benign disease refused an operation. An average of 17.5 days was recorded between PTD and operation, with one exception: A 71-year-old female patient had an indwelling drainage catheter for 247 days for treatment of an obstructed choledochojejunostomy due to a known carcinoma of the head of the pancreas, and was submitted to a relaparotomy in a different hospital, where a hepaticojejunostomy was performed (death occurred 2 days after surgery).

Of 34 patients with malignant disease, four had radical operations (Whipple's operations in three cases, total pancreatectomy in one), 20 had palliative operations; and 10 were found on exploration to be inoperable, so that the procedure had to end as an exploratory laparotomy.

Table 7. Complications in 116 cases of PTD

Serious:	Death	0
	Intraperitoneal biliary leakage	3
	Subcapsular haematoma	1
	Massive haemobilia	2
Mild:	Fever (with rigours in some cases)	19
	Cholangitis (including infection of the drainage tract)	14
	Catheter obstruction	7
	Displacement	35

In seven cases the PTD was left in situ for a period even after the operation (up to 60 days after surgery) to relieve the biliodigestive anastomosis.

In the meantime, all 91 patients with malignant disease have died; the mean survival time after PTD (with or without subsequent operation) was about 75 days, with the exception of three patients who were especially long-lived: (a) A 39-year-old patient with an inoperable tumour (bile duct carcinoma) metastasising into the hepatoduodenal ligament and portal region of the liver survived for 1 year 1 month, with external drainage and hardly any adjustment in his daily routine, until death (probably suicide). (b) A 38-year-old patient with a biliary tract carcinoma lived for 1 year 6 months with PTD, and even rebuilt his house during that time. (c) A 57-year-old patient with an (already resected) inoperable adenocarcinoma in the hilus of the liver survived for 3 years 4 months with external drainage, continuing with his job and sporting activities until shortly before his death.

Besides the four patients in whom attempts at drainage were unsuccessful and who underwent immediate operation, there were six further cases of severe complications amongst the 116 PTD procedures. Owing to localised clinical symptoms, five patients were operated upon shortly after PTD: one had a subcapsular haematoma, one had severe haemobilia, and the other three had leakage of bile without progression to a biliary peritonitis in the interval before operation. It appears that obscure epigastric symptoms after PTD are an indication for early operation to prevent a situation arising in which life is endangered by such severe complications, particularly as these are often initially bland.

In the sixth case the complete dislocation of an indwelling drain inserted some time previously led to performance of a second PTD, shortly after which a severe haemorrhage into the biliary system occurred. As the bleeding could not be stopped even with administration of Konakion we decided to carry out transfemoral selective coeliacography. After identifying the bleeding point we superselectively embolised the feeding vessel. The bleeding stopped and the clots which had formed in the biliary system were completely dissolved by extensive washouts via the indwelling external drainage catheter. Meanwhile, this drainage system is functioning with no complications whatsoever.

Two patients underwent operation 1 day after PTD because they had pulled out their catheters. The need for operation in these cases cannot be attributed to the method.

Mild and easily managed complications (Table 7), such as febrile reactions (in isolated cases with rigours due to an endotoxic reaction), were observed in 19 cases, cholangitis with infection of the drainage tract in 14 cases, and clogging of the catheter in seven cases. Since the introduction of systematic antibiotic prophylaxis before PTD or any extensive manipulation of the PTD system, such as catheter changing, we have very seldom seen a febrile reaction; in addition, the overall incidence of this type of reaction appears to be lowered if the procedure is carried out less forcibly during the exchange of bile for NaCl solution or contrast medium. Cholangitis with infection of the drainage canal or the thoracic wall was almost always associated with unsatisfactory drainage to the exterior. Catheter obstructions were, without doubt, attributable to lack of supervision during drainage. To avoid this kind of trouble it is necessary to give detailed instructions to the patients who are managed as outpatients, their relatives and their family doctors regarding the correct care of the drain.

The most common problem was evidently displacement of the catheter (35 cases). In 28 of these cases the previous drainage canal could be probed and a new catheter inserted; seven other cases required a completely new PTD after previous PTC. In one case PTD was completely dispensed with, as the patient had considerable ascites which prevented any assessment of the degree of bile leakage. Along with too-early mobilisation, forced respiratory movements, coughing and sneezing, ascites also represents a high risk factor for PTD: owing to free fluid in the space between thoracic wall and liver even the normal respiratory movements are sufficient to cause dislodgement of the drainage catheter from the liver. It is therefore recommended in all cases of ascites that the ascites be tapped completely before PTD is performed and the Teflon tube left in situ over the drainage catheter to provide a reinforcement between the thoracic wall and the liver.

Mild haemobilia is frequently observed, but tends to cease after a few hours without further intervention.

7.1 Discussion of Results

As a rule, patients with untreated obstructive jaundice (irrespective of its benign or malignant aetiology) die within a short time. The main causes of this are liver insufficiency and cachexia, along with infections of the biliary tree and gastrointestinal haemorrhages. An effective biliary drainage procedure offers patients with a liver still capable of recovery a definite improvement of their symptoms (pruritis, loss of appetite, poor general condition) as well as prolonged survival. By means of PTD, we were able to achieve an improvement in symptoms in 90% of our patients. 41 of these patients who had inoperable malignancies, had a mean survival time after PTD of about 60 days: one patient survived 1 year 1 month with drainage, another 1 year 6 months, and a third 3 years 4 months. Considering the inoperability of the disease, this procedure is the only means of improving survival, and there is some potential for further improvement, if patients are sent for PTD at an earlier stage and if satisfactory after-care of the indwelling drain can be guaranteed. As a large number of our patients with PTD (about one-third) come from other hospitals, precise documentation is unfortunately lacking and complete evaluation of the procedure is not possible; also, in some cases drainage was managed unsatisfactorily owing to inadequate knowledge of the method.

By means of PTD, a marked improvement in operability was achieved in 29 patients with malignant disease: on average the bilirubin fell from 15.6 mg% (max. 31.5, min. 6.5) before PTD to 4.0 mg% (max. 16.1, min. 0.3) before operation. In contrast to the high-risk so-called first decompression operation (*Buckwalter* et al. 1965; *Feduska* et al. 1971; *Hertzberg* 1974), we have not had a single death with PTD, and have observed serious complications in only 3.7% of cases. As PTD is as effective as decompression by drainage operation while associated with lower complication rates, involvement of less apparatus and personnel, better patient tolerance, and absence of adhesions (which are otherwise likely at a second operation), PTD should always be regarded as the method of choice for preoperative biliary drainage.

In our collective the success rate for PTD lies around 97%. We consider the incidence of serious complications (4% in our group) quite acceptable considering that equivalent operations are associated with a mortality of 10%–33% (*Brooks* and *Cutebras* 1976; *Buckwalter* et al. 1965; *Feduska* et al. 1971; *Hertzberg* 1974; *Nekase* et al. 1977) and that PTD represents the only therapeutic alternative for many patients with malignancies (about 60% according to our material).

Serious vascular complications, as reported by *Tylen* et al. (1977) in 15% and by *Hoevels* et al. (1980 a) in as many as 32% of cases, only occurred in two of our cases (1.7%). Impressed by the high incidence of aneurysms, haematomas, and arterioportal fistulas after PTD quoted by these two authors we carried out angiographic and CT checks of the last five PTD patients after drainage: we did not find a single further case of any of the above-mentioned vascular complications. These varying results may be explained as follows:

1. *Tylen* et al. (1977) and *Hoevels* et al. (1978) prefer the use of a very rigid guide wire for the introduction of the drainage catheter, which causes much more trauma to the liver than the coaxial Teflon tube that we use.
2. *Tylen* et al. (1977) and *Hoevels* et al. (1978) have to apply more force during the introduction of the drainage catheter, as their lateral caudal approach dictates a less favourable angle to the large bile ducts than our lateral cranial approach (Fig. 33).

The most common complication in our patients was displacement, in keeping with other studies, but this became less frequent as our technique improved (use of pig-tail catheters in external drainage, use of plaster to fix the catheter to skin, and stitching the catheter to the plaster) and meticulous follow-up care (24–48 h bedrest after PTD) was introduced.

Compared with the rare serious complications, the mild complications of PTD might be better described as side-effects rather than real complications.

7.2 Influence of PTD on Surgical Procedure

The majority of patients with malignant biliary obstructions die within a year (*Brooks* and *Culebras* 1976; *Buckwalter* et al. 1965; *Crile* 1970; *Feduska* et al. 1971; *Hertzberg* 1974; *Nakase* et al. 1977; *Shapiro* 1975). The operative results are poor for

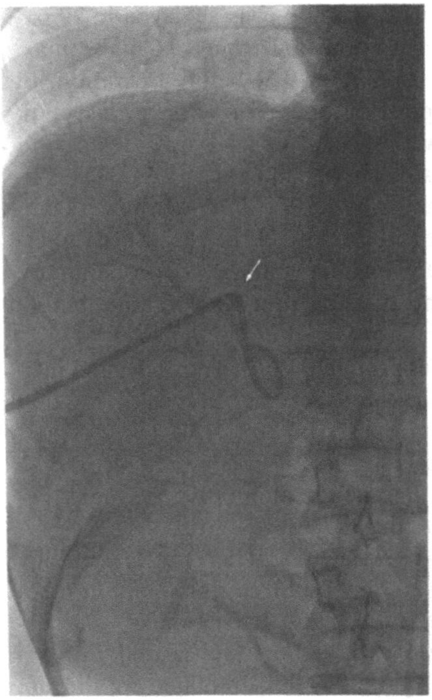

Fig. 33. Obstructive jaundice due to a metastasising gastric carcinoma in a 56-year-old patient. Unfavourable catheterisation direction associated with many complications: severe kinking of the drainage catheter in the liver at the site of entry to the central biliary system

all types of tumour; *Gudjonson* et al. (1978) quote a 5-year survival rate for pancreatic carcinoma of 0.4% (65 of 15,000 cases) and an average operative mortality of 22%. The average survival times after palliative bypass operation are around 5–7 months (*Brooks* and *Culebras* 1976; *Buckwalter* et al. 1965; *Crile* 1970; *Feduska* et al. 1971; *Hertzberg* 1974; *Nakase* et al. 1977; *Shapiro* 1975). After bypass operations, patients with bile duct carcinoma survive 14 months on average (*Harbin* and *Feruc-ci* 1980) and patients with papillary carcinoma, 22.7 months (*Nakase* et al. 1977) to 34 months (*Hertzberg* 1974).

Most cases are found to be inoperable at the time of operation due to extensive tumour growth, metastases or spread of tumour into the liver, so that the only possibility that can be entertained is palliative biliodigestive anastomosis.

The operative mortality of biliodigestive anastomosis lies between 10% and 33% (*Brooks* and *Culebras* 1976; *Buckwalter* et al. 1965; *Feduska* et al. 1971; *Hertzberg* 1974; *Nakase* et al. 1977). More extensive procedures are then associated with a much higher incidence of postoperative deaths with no improvement in survival (*Shamiyeh* 1974; *Treadwell* and *Hardin* 1976). In a high percentage of cases an exploratory laparotomy remains the only alternative (according to *Neugebauer* et al. 1979) about 40% in cases of bile duct carcinomas and about 30% with gallbladder carcinomas).

In our group, of 91 patients with malignant bile duct obstruction, 57 were initially inoperable; of 34 patients subjected to surgery, only four were suitable for radical operation (three of these patients died within 3 weeks after surgery), 20 patients had a biliodigestive anastomosis, and in 10 cases the operation was concluded after exploration.

The introduction of PTD as a routine method offers the surgeon the possibility of treating the patient without having to perform unnecessary, extensive and dangerous operations:

1. Exploratory laparotomy should be avoided in patients who are generally or locally inoperable, PTD should be employed instead. The survival rates improve as long as bile is drained, irrespective of whether a biliodigestive anastomosis or PTD provides drainage. (The postoperative mortality rate for a biliodigestive anastomosis lies between 10 and 33%, compared with less than 0.1% for PTD.)

2. PTD enables improved preoperative assessment of the operability of the tumour and of the feasibility of a biliodigestive anastomosis (this is due to better direct visualisation of the intra- and extrahepatic biliary system as well as the direct tumour biopsy through the catheter, which is possible during PTD as opposed to PTC).

The argument that tips the balance in favour of exploratory laparotomy for many surgeons is that there is still a remote chance of carrying out a curative procedure despite a preoperative diagnostic assessment of inoperability with regard to the tumour. *Gudjonsson* et al. (1978), for example, assess this chance at 0.4% with regard to the 5-year survival limit in a case of pancreatic surgical intervention, along with very high operative mortality, the surgeon is obliged – since the availability of PTD – to consider an elective operation with greater care than ever. In particular, cases such as the following should be prevented:

One of our patients, in whom a laterolateral choledochojejunostomy was obstructed by histologically proven carcinoma of the head of the pancreas, had a PTD for 247 days. The drainage was functioning so well that a surgeon began to doubt the histology and inoperability of the case. The patient was subjected to a repeat laparotomy, the histology was confirmed, and a terminolateral hepaticojejunostomy was constructed. The patient died of circulatory failure on the 2nd postoperative day.

3. In every case an operation to relieve obstruction is superseded by PTD to lower the high serum bilirubin levels before a second operation. In contrast to an operative decompression, the use and risks of PTD are unaffected by the level of serum bilirubin.

8 Effect of Biliary Obstruction and its Relief by PTD on the Portal Circulation

8.1 Hepatic Blood Flow and its Physiology

The blood supply to the liver consists of two vascular systems: in health about one-third is supplied by the hepatic artery and two-thirds by the portal vein (*Popper* and *Schaffner* 1957; *Ueda* 1962).

The hepatic artery supplies the liver parenchyma with oxygen (*Popper* and *Schaffner* 1957). Many researchers have expressed the view that the blood-supplying function of the hepatic artery is by no means vital (*Popper* et al. 1954). Of the blood flowing through the portal vein, 10%–35% comes from the spleen and 65%–90% from the mesenteric and gastric veins. According to *Popper* and *Schaffner* (1957) the portal venous blood is not necessary for the basic function of the liver, but is needed for the regeneration of liver tissue.

Blood from the hepatic artery and the portal vein flows through the perihilar plexus and the central veins into the hepatic veins. The low pressure in the intermittent flow of portal venous blood and the relatively high pressure of the blood flow from the hepatic artery into the liver is regulated by a complex system of inflow and outflow sphincters in the liver (*Elias* and *Sherrick* 1969; *Rappaport* 1960). Changes in the blood flow from the hepatic artery affect the portal vein and vice versa: an interruption in the portal venous supply causes vasodilatation of the hepatic artery, which in turn results in an increase in arterial blood flow by 50%–100% (*Andrews* 1968; *Burton-Opitz* 1911; *Fischer* and *Takacs* 1964; *Schenk* et al. 1960; *Schwiegk* 1932).

8.2 Portal Hypertension in the Presence of Obstructive Jaundice

Biliary obstruction causes an increase in presinusoidal resistance (*Reuter* and *Chuang* 1976), which leads to the development of portal hypertension if the obstruction persists with subsequent biliary cirrhosis. *Reuter* and *Chuang* (1976) demonstrated in animal experiments that complete obliteration of the common bile duct resulted in a presinusoidal intrahepatic block within 4 weeks, along with a decreased portal blood flow and a compensatory increased arterial blood flow. This increase in presinusoidal resistance precedes biliary cirrhosis (with the development of a sinusoidal and postsinusoidal block). Investigation of the vascular condition of the liver is therefore recommended in all patients with obstructive jaundice of any duration to assess the extent to which the blood flow has been affected. This can be done noninvasively by the method of quantitative liver perfusion scintigraphy developed by *Biersack* (1978).

8.2.1 Technique of Quantitative Liver Perfusion Scintigraphy

Technetium (Tc-99m)-pertechnetate (O_4^-) is used in the measurement of the arterial and portal venous fractions of the total hepatic blood flow. The quantity injected contains between 10 and 15 μCi. The total-body irradiation dose is between 0.01 and 0.02 mrad/μCi, the gonads receiving a similar dose. The critical organ is the thyroid gland, which has to be blocked by sodium perchlorate before the investigation is carried out. The patient's erythrocytes are labelled with Tc-99m-pertechnetate and are then reinjected as an "activity bolus" according to the Oldendorf technique (1965).

A time-activity curve with two peaks, as a result of the dual blood supply in health, can be imaged by a scintillation camera over the liver (Fig. 34) (for further details see *Biersack* 1978).

Biersack (1978) reports average values of 29.6% ± 1.4% for the arterial fraction of the total blood flow through normal liver, and 70.4% ± 1.4% for the portal venous fraction. In his patient group a median value for the arterial fraction of 74.7% ± 1.8% was obtained in the presence of portal hypertension, with a relative portal vascular volume of only 25.3% ± 1.8%. These values are also in keeping with the results quoted by *Zöckler* (1975), who reported a rise in arterial perfusion by about two-thirds of the total hepatic blood flow in the presence of portal hypertension.

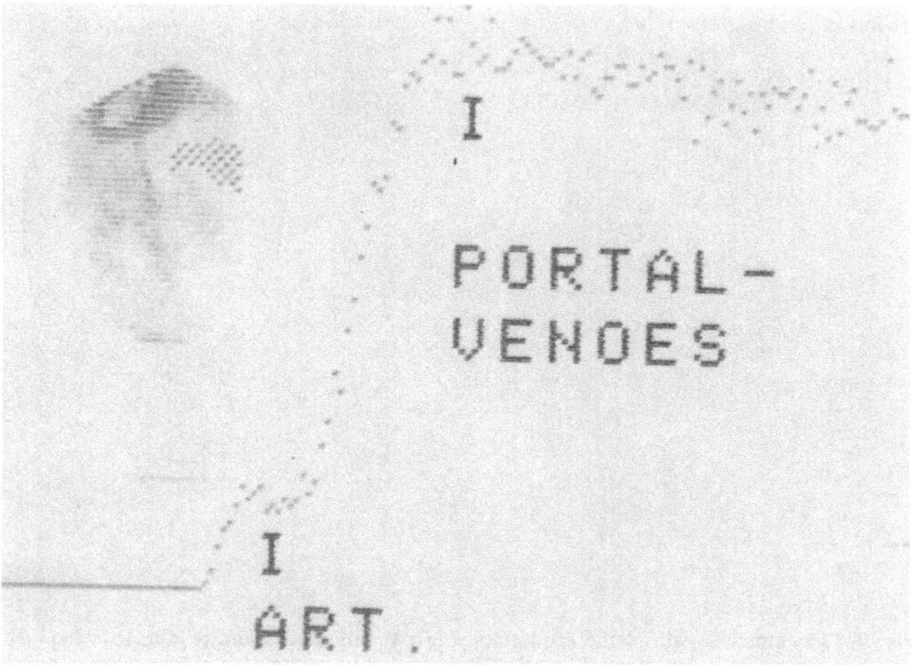

Fig. 34. Sequential hepatosplenic scintigraphy in health. Summation graph of the upper abdominal organs after an i.v. bolus of Tc-99 m. Histogram of the liver: impulse integral of the arterial phase, 1094 counts = 10.5%; impulse integral of the portal-venous phase, 9109 counts = 89.5%

8.2.2 Our Own Results

Quantitative liver perfusion scintigraphy was carried out by the method described above immediately before PTD in a 70-year-old patient with obstructive jaundice of some weeks' standing (Fig. 35). The initial serum bilirubin was 21.9 mg%; previous CT and ultrasound investigations had shown an intrahepatic biliary system dilated to 1.25 cm at the most; no parenchymal changes suggesting cirrhosis were demonstrable. Liver perfusion scintigraphy showed that 92.0% of the hepatic blood flow was of arterial and 8.0% of portal venous origin. After only 14 days of biliary drainage by PTD, when the bilirubin level had fallen to 8.0 mg%, the liver perfusion scintigraphy was repeated (Fig. 36); the arterial contribution to the liver blood flow was 46%, the remaining 54% being of portal venous origin. Similar results with this investigation were achieved in five of a total of 10 patients.

8.2.3 Discussion

Our observations of portal hypertension in our patients with complete obstruction of the common bile duct for some length of time without evidence of liver cirrhosis agree with the results of Reuter's experiments with animals (*Reuter* and *Chuang*

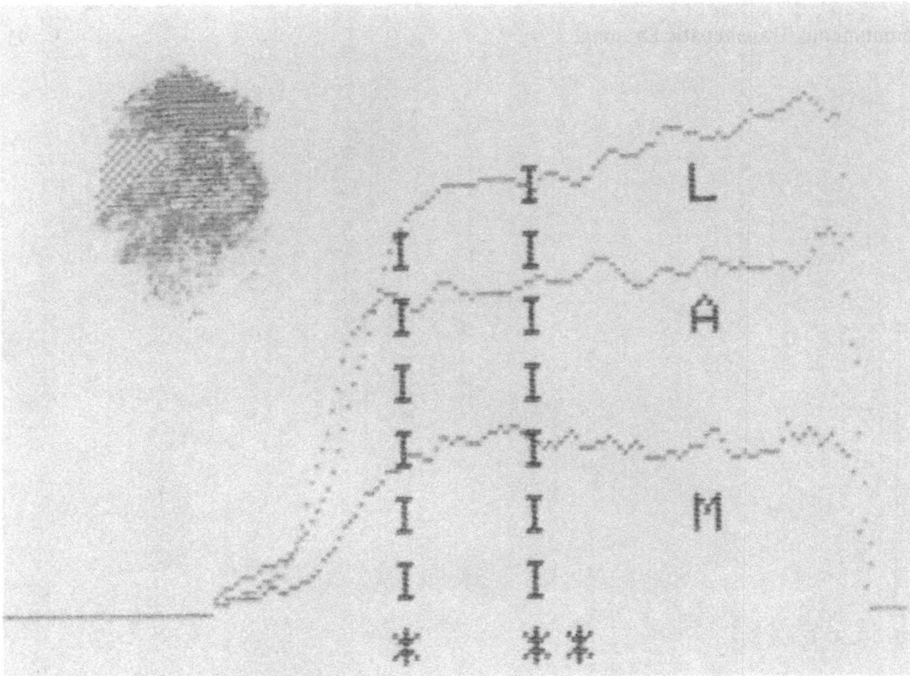

Fig. 35. Sequential hepatosplenic scintigraphy in patients with jaundice due to a high obstruction (serum bilirubin about 30 mg%). Marked portal hypertension before relief of biliary obstruction by PTD. Relative arterial blood flow in the liver, 92.0% (≙ 3724 counts); relative portal venous blood flow in the liver, 8.0% (≙ 323 counts)

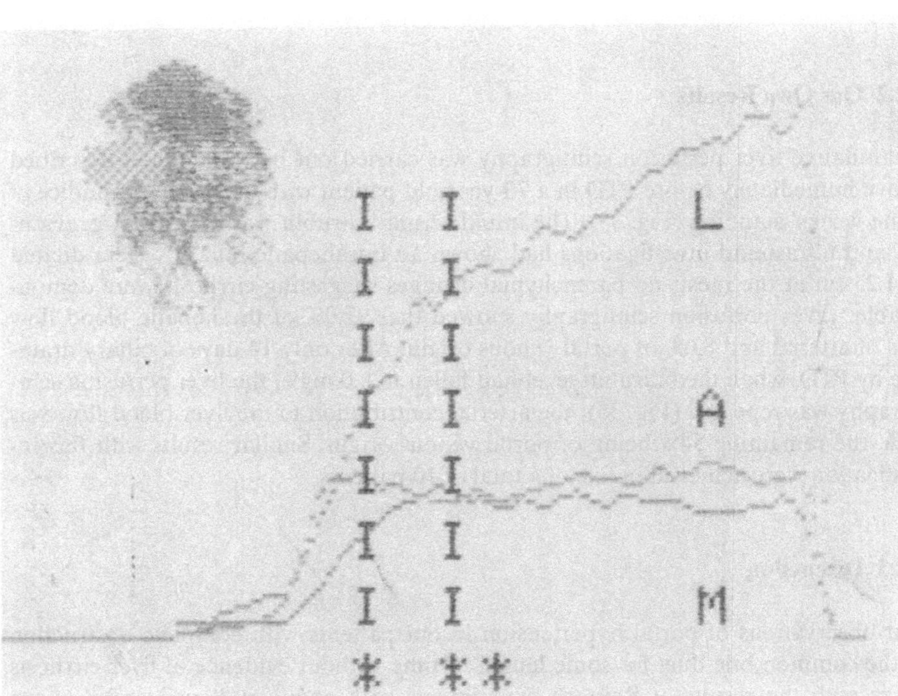

1976). The portal hypertension tended to improve markedly after biliary drainage, which indicates its reversibility in such cases.

Investigations in man to elucidate the improved vascular situation in the liver after drainage of the biliary system and to clarify the association between biliary obstruction and portal hypertension have been equally scarce. It is possible that the improvement in portal hypertension after decompression of the biliary system represents a decisive factor for the general improvement in the operability of these patients.

PTD in association with quantitative liver perfusion scintigraphy offers for the first time a means of investigating in man the relationships between the duration and extent of biliary obstruction and the development of portal hypertension, as well as its regression after biliary drainage.

9 Therapeutic Implications of an Indwelling Drainage Catheter

Relief of biliary obstruction is certainly not the only therapeutic use of PTD; it also facilitates such procedures as percutaneous transhepatic antegrade manipulations, e.g., crushing stones or dilating strictures in the biliary tree.

9.1 Antegrade Stone Crushing and Extraction

In up to 5% (*Burhenne* 1974) of cases operated on for stones in the biliary duct one or more concretions are left in the common hepatic bile duct, making a second or third operation necessary. These repeat laparotomies are associated with mortality of between 3% and 11% (*Hess* 1977; *Smith* et al. 1969). *Burhenne* (1972) in the United States has developed a method for nonoperative percutaneous extraction of concretions from the common bile duct and the larger biliary ducts.

Stones in the hepatic bile duct and the larger biliary channels can be crushed and extracted in a similar fashion via PTD. Antegrade crushing of stones in the hepatic bile duct is accomplished by exchanging the catheter for a catheter fitted with a basket for stone extraction (Fig. 37). The concretions are grasped by the basket and crushed by applying the technique described by *Burhenne* (1972). Stones, or fragments of stones, that do not have a diameter much greater than the lumen of the drainage channel can be completely removed by the stone-extracting basket or can be pushed distally through the stenosis.

On the basis of a similar case of our own (Fig. 38), we consider this method a practical and simple extension of PTD which is associated with few complications;

Fig. 36. Sequential hepatosplenic scintigraphy in the same patient as in Fig. 35 after relief of the biliary obstruction by means of PTD. Significant improvement of the portal hypertension. Relative arterial blood flow in the liver, 46.0% (≙ 1486 counts); relative portal venous flow in the liver, 54.0% (≙ 1785 counts). *L* = histogram of the liver; *A* = histogram of the aorta; *M* = histogram of the spleen; +, arterial phase of the blood flow in the liver; + +, portal venous phase of the blood flow in the liver

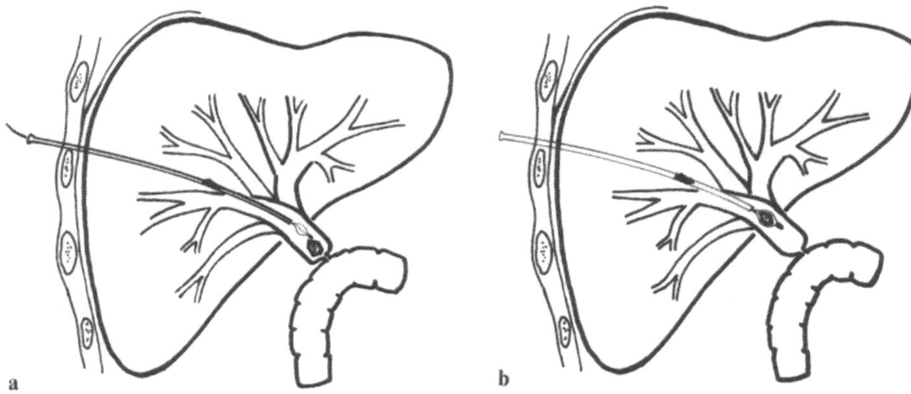

Fig. 37 a, b. Technique of antegrade percutaneous transhepatic stone crushing and extraction. **a** Exchanging the external percutaneous transhepatic drainage catheter for a catheter with a stone-extracting basket; **b** Grasping the biliary calculus with the stone-extracting basket in the bile duct to crush or extract the calculus

this has only recently been confirmed by *Günther* et al. (1982). It is recommended that manipulations such as stone crushing or extraction, as well as the dilating procedure described below, are postponed until the drain has been established for several weeks and the drainage tract is lined with connective tissue, to allow easier catheter exchange and subsequent reinsertion of a drainage catheter.

9.2 Antegrade Dilatation of Benign Stenoses of the Common Bile Duct

In radiology percutaneous transluminal dilatation of stenoses has so far been applied in transluminal angioplasty (*Dotter* 1980). This technique can also be applied in the antegrade dilatation of benign strictures of the common bile duct.

A guide wire is used to exchange the PTD catheter by the Seldinger technique for a Grüntzig balloon dilatation catheter. To protect the drainage canal and the balloon catheter, this should be carried out with a Teflon tube. Under X-ray screening the balloon of the dilatation catheter is positioned exactly in the region of the stricture (Fig. 39; in this case in the anastomotic stricture), and the stenosis is then slowly dilated pneumatically until the balloon is inflated to its maximum and can be moved freely through the stricture.

We performed a percutaneous transhepatic antegrade dilatation of a hepaticojejunostomy stricture in a patient who has now been free of symptoms for 4 years and 3 months without any signs of recurrence of the obstructive jaundice or of cholangitis. A recent check by liver sequence scintigraphy showed no abnormality of bile flow. In a second case, several attempts at dilating an anastomotic stricture were unsuccessful because it was caused by external tumour compression and was not a purely benign cicatricial stricture, as became apparent later.

Molnar and *Strockum* (1978) have published reports of dilatation of benign strictures after choledochoenterostomies; nine of 13 dilatation attempts were successful. Up to a period of 7 years after dilatation there were no recurrences of jaun-

Fig. 38a, b. A 65-year-old female patient had frequent recurrent episodes of cholangitis and development of a biliary cirrhosis over a period of 8 years. A hepaticojejunostomy had been constructed earlier during bilious peritonitis after a cholecystectomy for cholelithiasis. Now clinical evidence of obstructive jaundice. **a** High degree of stenosis in the hepaticojejunostomy, with additional obstruction at the hepatic confluence due to a large impacted biliary calculus. **b** Visualisation of the fragmented calculi further above the stricture after repeated percutaneous transhepatic antegrade stone crushing with the DORMIA biliary stone-extracting basket. In addition, external PTD has been converted to internal PTD

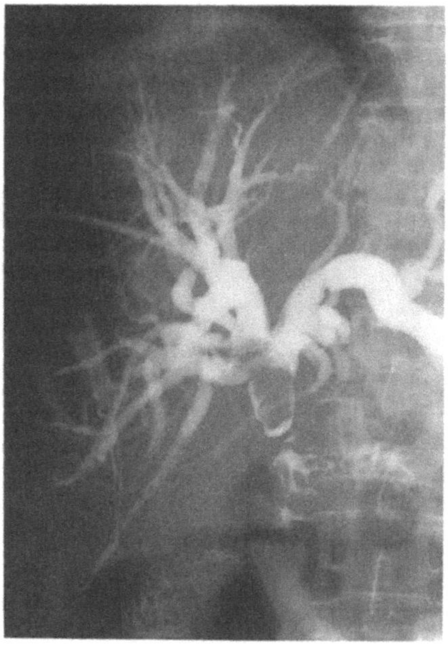

a

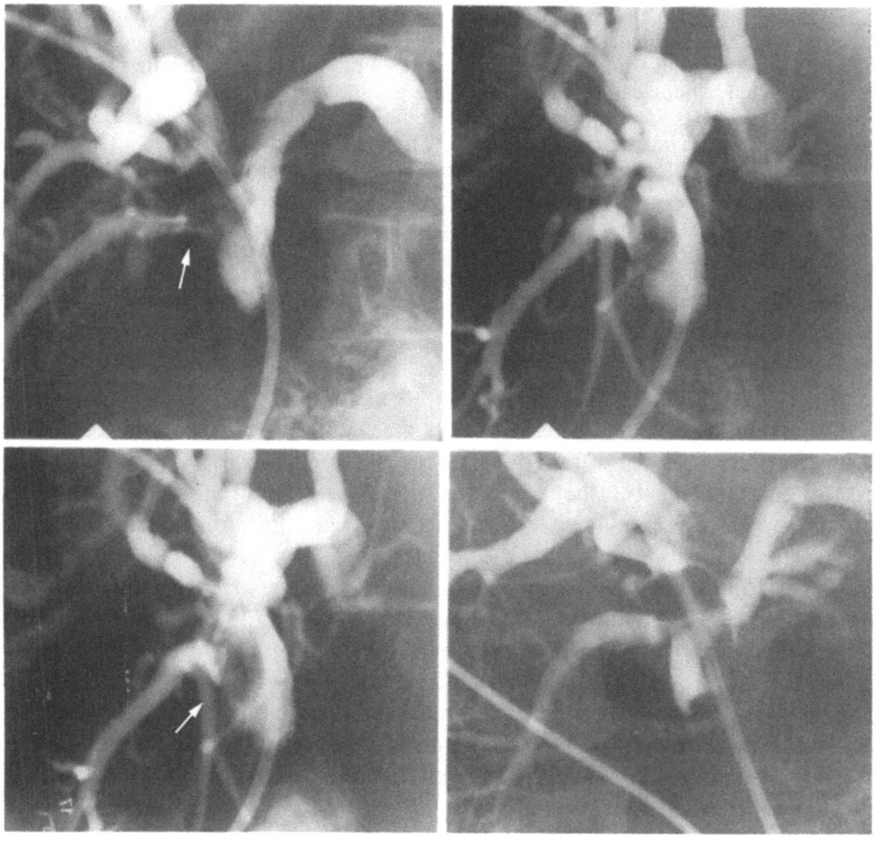

b

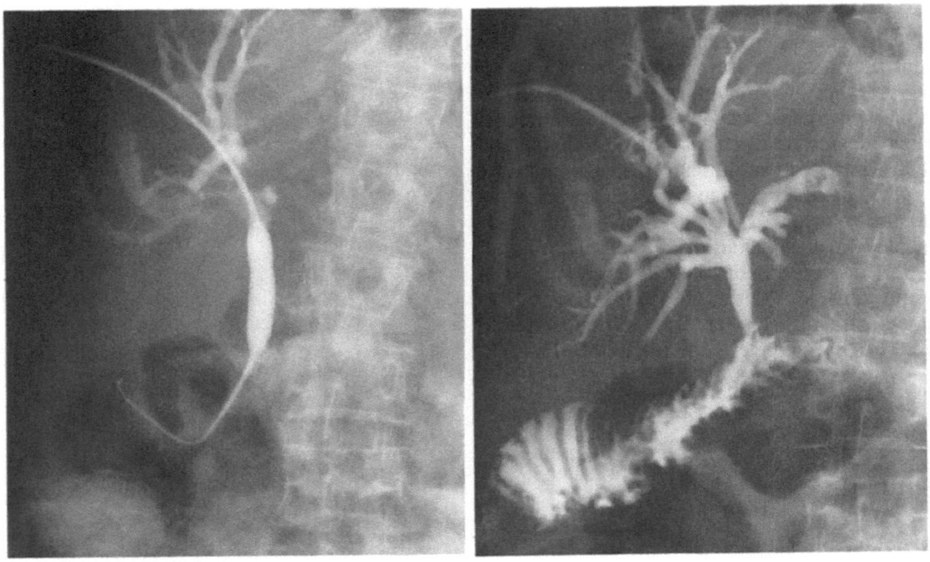

a

Fig. 39 a, b. The same patient as in Fig. 38. Percutaneous antegrade transhepatic dilatation of the anastomotic stricture. After 4 weeks continuous internal PTD, we exchanged the drainage catheter for a balloon dilatation catheter and carried out pneumatic dilatation of the stricture. **a** Contrast filled balloon catheter dilated within the anastomotic stricture. The pneumatic dilatation was repeated 4 times at weekly intervals, the final procedure involving the use of a balloon catheter with a maximum diameter of 9 mm. **b** Anastomosis dilated to a diameter of 8 mm. (N.B. Air bubbles in the biliary system, especially on the left)

dice or ascending cholangitis. Not a single case exhibited such complications as bilious peritonitis or sub- or intrahepatic abscesses.

The percutaneous transhepatic procedure thus offers a real alternative to operative treatment of benign anastomotic strictures, bearing in mind the operative difficulties caused by adhesions around the operating site and the high recurrence rate [25%–35% (*Smith* 1964)]. Of course, a lowering of the recurrence rate cannot be expected. Percutaneous transhepatic dilatation, however, is easy and can be performed repeatedly; it is well tolerated by the patient and associated with few complications; and the option of an operation remains open.

The dilatation procedure can be applied to anastomotic strictures as well as benign stenoses in the region of the common bile duct or of one of the hepatic bile ducts if these are the cause of the patient's symptoms. Dilatation is not indicated if external or internal drainage fails to bring about a fall in the bilirubin level after 2–3 weeks of drainage.

9.3 Localised Radiotherapy with PTD

In addition to the possibility of direct manipulations, PTD also offers a means of relieving biliary obstruction by localised percutaneous radiotherapy in the portal region of the liver or around the hepatic bile duct.

Until recently it was generally believed that bile duct and gallbladder carcinomas and pancreatic carcinomas were resistant to radiotherapy (*Moerkel* 1973). This was an error based on the observation that adenocarcinomas in toto respond less well to radiotherapy than squamous cell carcinomas (*Hanna* et al. 1978) and that survival times used to be too short, owing to progressive jaundice, to identify the effect of radiotherapy (*Hashmonai* et al. 1980). Meanwhile, several reports on radiotherapy of gallbladder, bile duct and pancreatic carcinomas have appeared; as a rule, the number of case reports is very small and the techniques of irradiation differ considerably.

9.3.1 Results Reported in the Literature

As far back as 1935, *Walters* and *Olson* treated a patient with an inoperable carcinoma of the papilla intraoperatively with interstitially implanted radium (140 mgeh), and in 1940 *Lam* (1940) treated another three patients with gallbladder carcinomas in the same way. *Ariel* and *Pack* (1960) applied infusions of iodine-123-Rose Bengal to their patients with inoperable biliary duct carcinomas. Most groups of workers irradiated the biliary duct region with telecobalt units over opposing ventral-dorsal erect fields with doses between 10 and 70 Gy (*Friedland* 1971; *Green* et al. 1973; *Hudgins* and *Meoz,* to be published; *Krain* 1972; *Moossa* et al. 1975; *Terblanche* et al. 1972; *Terblanche* and *Lower* 1973; *Treadwell* and *Hardin* 1976; *Van Heerden* et al. 1967; *Vaittenen* 1970). *Kopelson* et al. (1977), *Smorow* (1977) and *Dobelbower* et al. (1980) used photon radiation with an energy between 4 MeV and 45 MeV in a total dose up to 70 Gy (in about 1.8-Gy fractions).

The efficacy of radiotherapy in carcinomas of gallbladder, biliary ducts, and pancreas is now established. Despite the small number of only 11 patients treated, *Pipelich* and *Lambert* (1978) consider radiotherapy to be very effective in the treatment of bile duct carcinomas, not only in addition to surgery, but also as a treatment in its own right in cases of locally limited operability where a radical operation is precluded: in five patients treated by radiation only the survival times were 3 months, over 6 months, 8 months, 17 months, and 26 months.

According to *Dobelbower* et al. (1980) the results of precisely localised, high-dose radiotherapy in cases of pancreatic carcinomas no longer suitable for radical operation were similar to operative results obtained in patients in whom radical resection of tumour was possible: the 1-year survival rate in their patient collective was 49%.

The exact extent to which radiotherapy is effective in malignant obstructive jaundice can only be assessed in the future, after the possibility of biliary decompression by PTD with few complications has been realised and patients no longer have to face early death from obstructive jaundice. PTD offers a simultaneous means of checking the effects of irradiation directly at the target organ: a complete tumorous obstruction of the biliary system can regress to a stenosis, or a stricture can be dilated to a duct of normal diameter.

9.3.2 Our Own Results with Percutaneous Telecobalt Irradiation During Indwelling PTD

In four patients with inoperable malignancies two cases of gallbladder carcinoma, one of biliary duct carcinoma, and one of distant metastasis to the hepatoduodenal ligament), we instituted PTD and then administered percutaneous telecobalt therapy over a ventral erect field (Table 8). The irradiation fields were localised after visualisation of the biliary system via PTD with radiological screening. The tumour depth was assumed to be between 5 and 9 cm; at this time CT-orientated radiation planning was not yet available. In three patients the total radiation dose was around 30 Gy, in one other patient around 40 Gy of the assumed tumour depth.

During radiotherapy two patients showed opening of the tumour obstruction in the hepatic bile ducts, so that the external drainage could be converted to internal drainage (Fig. 40). After completing radiotherapy, one patient exhibited partial, filiform patency of the tumour obstruction which, however, was not sufficient for conversion to internal drainage. In the patient irradiated with the higher dose, no evidence has yet been observed of any widening of the common bile duct stenosis. The only side-effects of irradiation were loss of appetite and fatigue.

Three of the irradiated patients have since died (mean survival time 185 days); one female patient is still alive 130 days after PTD. In one case the cause of death was the recurrence of obstructive jaundice with a nonfunctioning PTD, unfortunately not referred back to us for correction.

9.3.3 Discussion of Results

The opening of the tumorous obstructions in the two irradiated cases must be considered without any doubt as an effect of the radiotherapy. It is not possible, however, to assess whether the longer-than-average survival times are due to the effect of the irradiation.

To avoid complications, the dose we used was very low compared with *Kopelson* et al.'s (1977) recommendation of a dose of 45–50 Gy over a period of 4–5 weeks in connection with the effect of irradiation on adenocarcinomas originating at other sites (Committee for Radiation Oncology Studies 1976). On the other hand, *Green* et al. (1973) report on a patient in whom no evidence of tumour was found at autopsy after irradiation of a biliary duct carcinoma with 20 Gy.

The general side-effects were significantly less severe than expected. This can be attributed to the low dose and the care taken to involve as little of the liver parenchyma in the radiation field as possible, and certainly also to the relief of the biliary system obstruction by the PTD.

Fig. 40 a–c. 50-year-old patient with metastases from a vaginal carcinoma into the hepatoduodenal ligament. **a** PTD reveals highly localised, complete occlusion of the common bile duct through which an internal drainage catheter has been introduced into the duodenum. **b** Opening up of the obstruction and opacification of the stenosis caused by metastases immediately after telecobalt radiotherapy (direct ventral erect field, 30 Gy in 3 weeks). **c** Definite regression of the malignant stenosis 3 months after completion of the course of radiotherapy

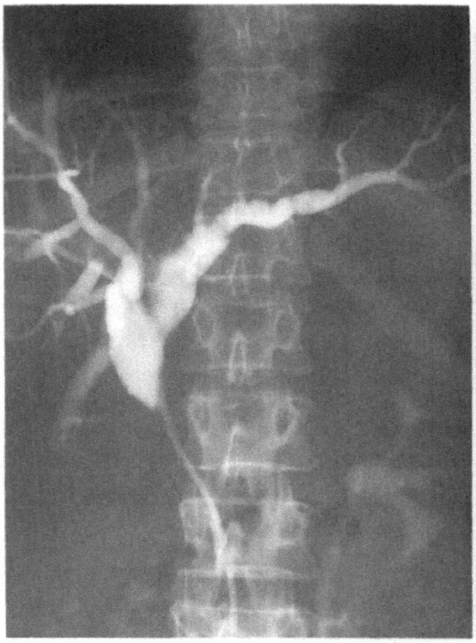
a

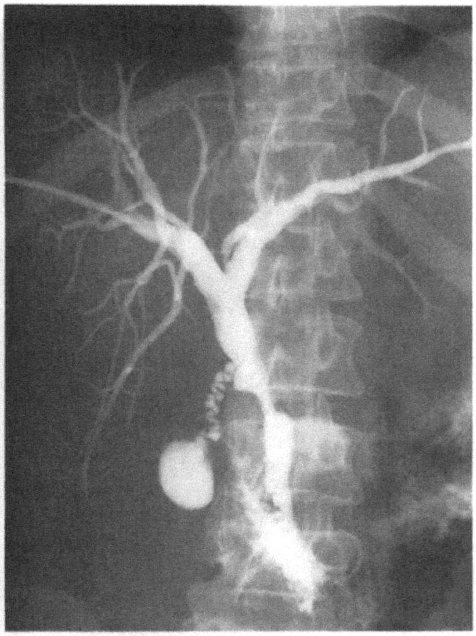
c

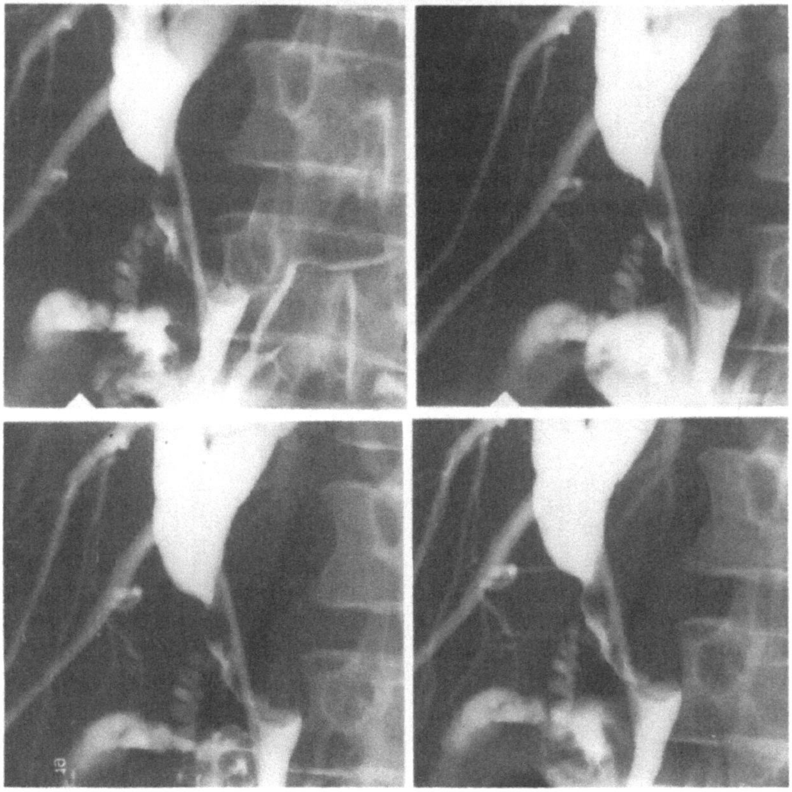
b

Table 8. Percutaneous radiotherapy with PTD

				Irradiation data						
Patient	Age and sex	Type of tumour	Local findings (operation)	Field size (cm)	Focussing depth (cm)	Gy fractions	Total dose (Gy)	Local effects of therapy	Survival (days)	Cause of death
1	66 years F	Gallbladder carcinoma	Locally inoperable (probataria 18 days after PTD)	6× 8	5	4×2.10	29.4	Filiform patency of the obstructed common hepatic bile duct	180	Liver metastases
2	50 years F	Metastases from vaginal carcinoma	Inoperable (probataria 34 days after PTD)	6×10	9	4×1.50	30.0	Regression of tumorous stricture (internal drainage)	287	Generalised malignant cachexia
3	73 years M	Gallbladder carcinoma	Inoperable (construction of a Kehr drainage system)	10×10	8	4×1.37	30.25	Opening up of the malignant stricture (internal drainage)	90	Recurrence of obstructive jaundice
4	57 years F	Gallbladder carcinoma	Inoperable (cholecystectomy 15 months previously)	7× 7	5	5×1.95	39.8	No change in malignant stenosis	130 to date	

It appears to us that the successes of radiotherapy with indwelling PTD presented here are sufficiently encouraging to allow a generous assessment of the indications for this procedure.

9.3.4 Discussion of Irradiation Technique

One aim of radiation therapy in the treatment of malignant obstructive jaundice is permanent widening of the biliary duct stenoses or opening up of the obstruction, and the other is the most extensive devitalisation of tumour tissue possible. As these carcinomas frequently exhibit localised growth, they are particularly suitable for high-dose localised radiotherapy. In percutaneous irradiation, however, the ratio of actual target volume to inadvertently irradiated volume is very infavourable; the latter includes critical organs such as intestine, liver, and kidney. As for gynaecological tumours, the optimal radiotherapy here would also consist in a combination of percutaneous high-voltage therapy and precisely aimed small-space contact irradiation. The advantage of this contact irradiation lies in the high dose in the region of the source and the steep rate of dose reduction with increasing distance from the source.

Percutaneous transhepatic drainage proves an intraductal means of approach to the tumour such as is found with gynaecological carcinomas. By making use of the drainage channel we have developed an intraductal radiotherapy with the afterloading technique.

9.4 Intraductal Irradiation with the Afterloading Technique

The prerequisite for intraductal irradiation is PTD of some duration which has allowed the drainage canal in the chest wall and liver to become lined with connective tissue enabling repeated catheter changes to be performed painlessly and conveniently.

9.4.1 Instruments and Radiation Source

The instruments needed for radiation (Fig. 41) are:

- Afterloading device (in this case Gamma-Med II from Isotopen-Technik Sauerwein (1976)
- Flexible polyethylene applicator probe with closed end, 25 mm in length (OD 3 mm, ID 2 mm)
- Teflon tube, 17.5 cm in length (OD 3.5 mm)
- Thick-walled rigid Oedmann-Ledin catheter, approx. 30 cm in length (OD 2.8 mm)
- J guide wire
- Simulation cable, approx. 30 cm in length (OD 2 mm).

Normally the afterloading device is used for contact and short-distance irradiation of gynaecological tumours: the source, soldered to a metal cable, is guided electromotively from the shielding container through a polyethylene tube to the

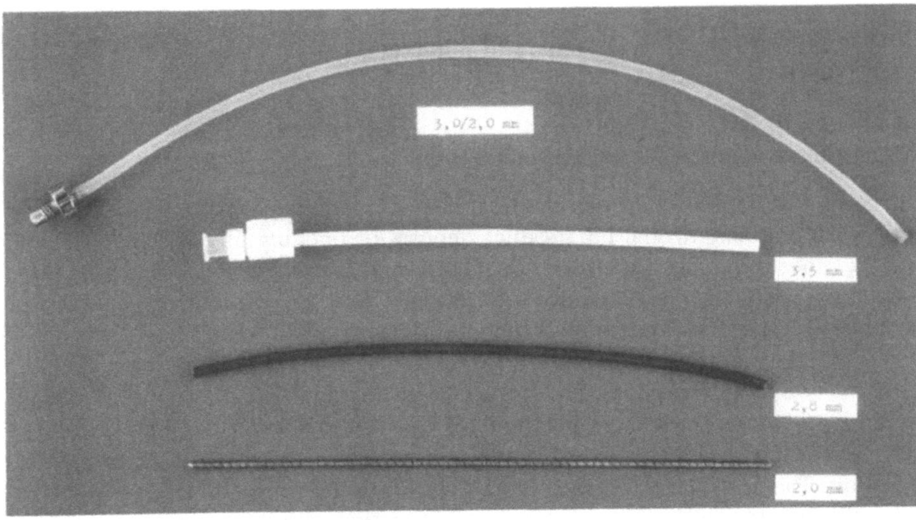

Fig. 41. Instruments needed for afterloading irradiation

probe that has been placed in the tumour. After expiration of the irradiation time the source is retracted to the shielding. We use an iridium-192 source, which, due to its high specific activity (approx. 600 Ci/g), is particularly suitable for our purpose. The source is almost punctiform with diameters of 1 mm (cylindrical), and has an initial activity of 10 Ci. The source is enclosed by a 0.4-mm stainless steel covering. The small external measurements of source and covering allow smooth passage through the applicator probe (possible with an ID of 2 mm) that we have developed.

The high dose rate of iridium allows short irradiation times (a few minutes only) and thus shortens the treatment time for the patient and the application of the applicator probe, which impedes bile drainage. Due to the short irradiation time the reproducibility of the dose distribution at the target is guaranteed.

9.4.2 Preparation of the Patient

For the percutaneous transhepatic introduction of the closed-end application probe into the biliary system up to the tumour obstruction or through the tumour stenosis, a Teflon tube with as thin walls as possible must be used, which can then be used coaxially for external splinting (Fig. 42). As this thin-walled Teflon tube is easily compressed and bent, the drainage catheter is first exchanged by the Seldinger technique over an indwelling introducing wire for a thick-walled, rigid catheter with an external diameter of about 2.8 mm, over which the tube can then be advanced into the biliary system up to the site of the tumour. After removal of the catheter and the introducing wire, the application probe is introduced with ease up to the obstructing tumour or through the tumour stenosis. The free movement of the radiation source lying intracorporeally in the application probe is checked by advancing it to the end of the probe and then retracting a simulating cable, which possesses the same external dimension and pliability as the cable with the radiation source.

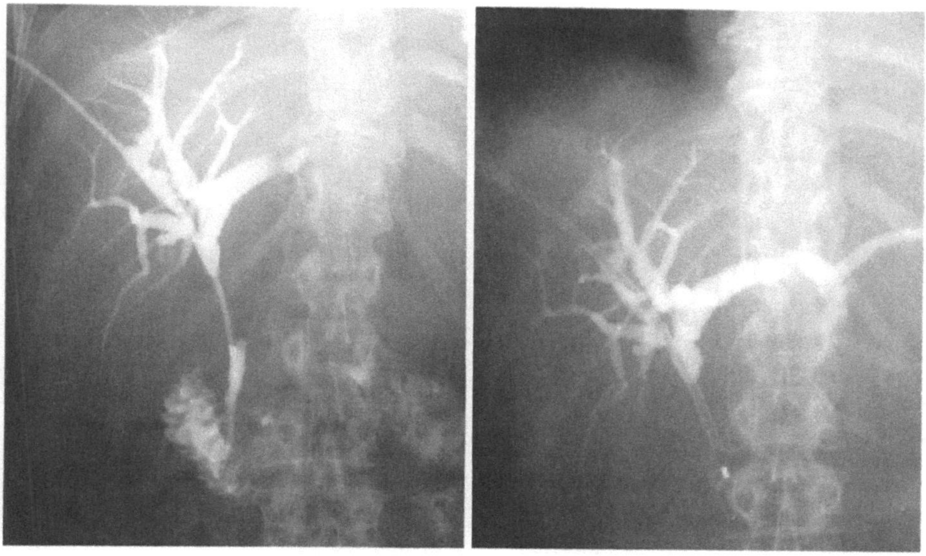

b

Fig. 42 a, b. Inoperable gallbladder carcinoma in a 57-year-old female patient. Preparation for intraductal radiotherapy by afterloading technique via the indwelling internal PTD drain. **a** Internal PTD in situ, with the catheter tip lying in the common bile duct distal to the tight malignant stricture. **b** Applicator probe lying in the Teflon tube. The radio-opaque, closed free end of the probe lies in the distal part of the common bile duct

When an indwelling PTD system has been in place for some time this dilatation of the drainage canal and the insertion of the applicator probe prove quite uncomplicated and painless, so that premedication and local anaesthesia of the chest wall or liver are unnecessary.

9.4.3 Planning and Administration of Radiotherapy

With the help of a computer program, the desired isodose distribution is calculated according to the site, size, and extent of the tumour. The program determines the parameters needed for guiding the afterloading, e.g. commencement and termination of the irradiation and exposure time of the applicator at the target points and the control points. When the isodose pictures calculated by computer agree with the isodose distribution decided on, irradiation is started.

In the patient we irradiated by this technique, the dose desired and achieved at a point 1 cm from the application probe was 15 Gy directly at the applicator per session, with a smooth isodose distribution curve in the computer-calculated isodose picture (Fig. 43). After a preceding percutaneous irradiation with cobalt-60 (38.5 Gy) and subsequent irradiation by the after-loading procedure on three occasions the tumour stenosis did not show any signs of opening up. The patient reacted to irradiation by the after-loading procedure with a short bout of nausea and vomiting.

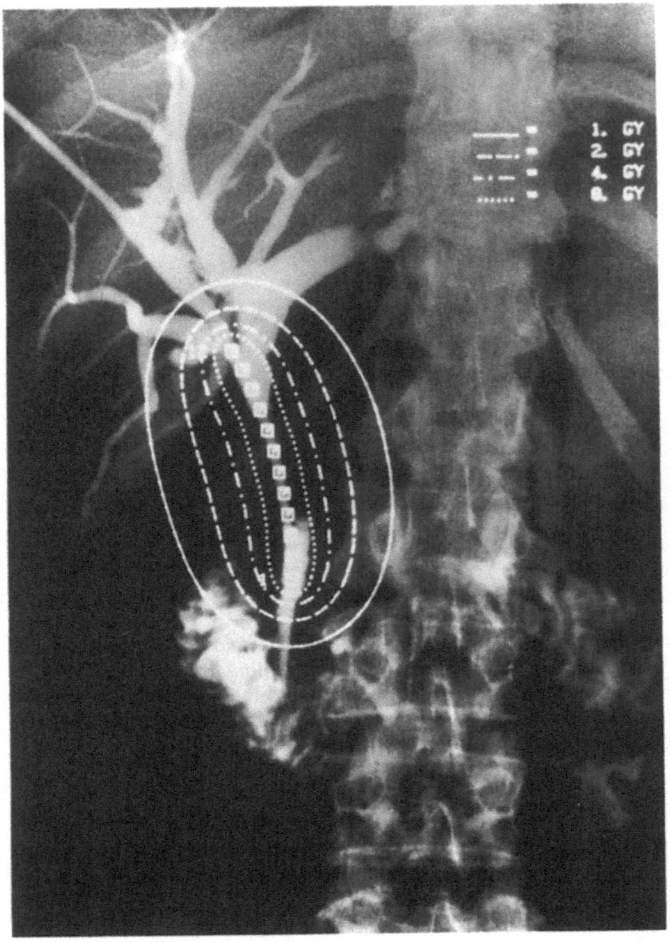

Fig. 43. Inoperable gallbladder carcinoma in a 57-year-old patient (see Fig. 42b). Computerised isodose distribution of the irradiation of the bile duct stenosis by iridium-192 afterloading

9.4.4 Discussion

The technical procedure involved in irradiating tumorous biliary duct obstructions has been developed to the stage where all patients with indwelling percutaneous biliary drainage accomplished according to the method described above can be irradiated.[2] The necessary spatial isodose distributions, particularly with complete tumour obstructions, can be optimised with the aid of a computer program and carried out with the Gamma-Med II. Experience with determination of the necessary dose for contact therapy, alone or in combination with percutaneous irradiation, and any complications has not yet been published.

Iwasaki et al. (1977) give a growth-inhibiting and thus complication-free dose of 30 Gy for percutaneous irradiated biliary duct and gallbladder carcinomas. *Todoroki* et al. (1976) irradiated the liver hili of rabbits percutaneously in single sessions with 30–50 Gy without observing any severe progressive damage to biliary ducts, vessels, or liver; all rabbits survived for 10 months. In contrast, a single session of irradiation with 100 Gy caused severe progressive vascular changes leading to the death of all rabbits within 10 months.

Radiation therapy by the afterloading procedure via PTD[3] offers, for the first time, the possibility of applying high doses directly to biliary duct and gallbladder carcinomas with a readily reproducible radiation geometry in the target volume, thus providing a means of gathering the experience so far lacking regarding the efficacy and complication rates of radiotherapy of these cancers, as well as improving their treatment.

10 Long-Term Biliary Drainage

The duration of PTD possible with an indwelling system is unlimited, as far as the method is concerned. In practice, however, the duration of PTD depends either on the operation performed after achieving a fall in bilirubin in the case of benign obstructions (i.e., if direct treatment by means of PTD in the form of pneumatic dilatation or stone extraction is precluded) or, in the case of a malignant aetiology, on the extent of the tumour at the time of examination or drainage, as well as on the general condition of the patient and the aggressiveness of tumour growth.

In a small number of cases long-term indwelling drainage associated with particular problems has been reported. The longest duration for PTD has so far been reported by *Nakayama* et al. (1978) to be 2 years 1 month. We have observed three drainage systems over a period of about 1 year in one case, of about 1 year 6 months in a second case, and of about 3 years 4 months in the third case.

Some of the special problems of long-term PTD have been described in association with short-term drainage; they can be classified in four groups.

10.1 Catheter Breakage, Obstruction, and Displacement

We ourselves have never observed a catheter breakage, but this is described by *Molnar* and *Stockum* (1974). The constant respiratory movements are said to cause fatigue of the material, with subsequent breakage of the catheter. *Molnar* and *Stockum* (1974), rather like *Ring* et al. (1979), therefore recommend changing the catheter every 2–3 months even if function is still good. In our experience one should wait until there is a real indication, e.g., obstruction, dislocation or inflammation.

Catheter obstruction presents no great problems as long as it is due to encrustation, which can be easily remedied by the insertion of an introducing wire. The best

3 After development of our own intraductal irradiation technique was complete, a similar technique developed by *Fletcher* et al. (1981) and *Herskovic* et al. (1981) became known to us. It will be possible to assess its effect on the biliary system directly by fibre-endoscopic examinations with biopsies (see Sect. 11.3)

way of avoiding encrustation of the catheter is naturally regular flushing, up to twice daily, with repeated applications of 10–15 ml physiological NaCl solution. In these washouts a minimum pressure has to be maintained to ensure good flushing of the side-holes.

As with short-term indwelling catheters, frequent catheter displacements must be expected with long-term indwelling drains; however, as with long-term catheters there is generally a granulated transparenchymal drainage tract through the chest wall and liver. Reinsertion of the catheter is generally possible without any difficulties. In a few isolated cases it is not possible to make out the drainage tract even after injecting contrast medium through the opening in the chest wall and opacifying the drainage channel in the liver; in these cases a renewed PTC with subequent PTD is necessary (Fig. 44).

To keep the difficulties of displacement to a minimum, we instruct our patients and insist that they return to our institute as soon as the catheter slips out of the chest wall or the bile flow stops; as the catheter usually does not slip out of the liver and chest wall simultaneously, reinsertion is considerably easier at this stage than when the catheter has been completely removed.

10.2 Biliary Leakage Around the Catheter, Fistula Formation, and Inflammation of the Biliary System, Skin and Thoracic Wall

As a rule, the occurrence of biliary leakage (as with short-term drainage) reflects impaired drainage through the tubing or dilatation of the drainage channel compared with the external diameter of the catheter, which is often the result of necrosis in the liver parenchyma around the catheter and an inflammatory process.

The formation of fistulas in the thoracic wall or between chest wall and liver and inflammation in the catheter tract usually cause no further symptoms. As a rule, bile leakages disappear when the catheter is exchanged for a thicker one (our maximum

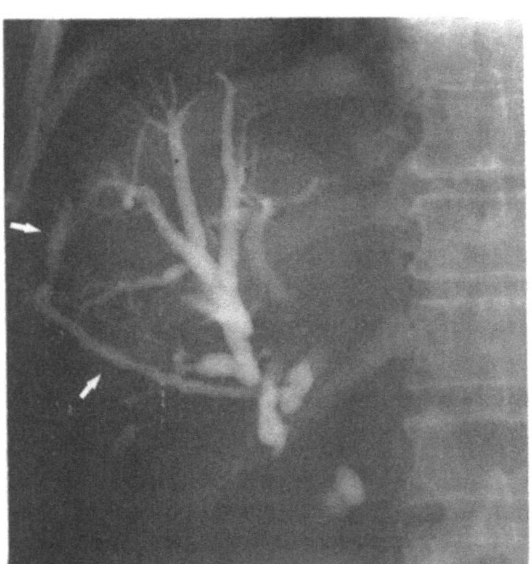

Fig. 44. Distal obstruction of the common bile duct caused by a carcinoma of the head of the pancreas in a 62-year-old female patient. After a complete catheter displacement a new PTC was necessary, as it was not possible to reinsert a new catheter in the old drain tract. Retrograde filling via repeated PTC allowed opacification of the old drainage canal in the chest wall and liver along with a fistula between liver and chest wall

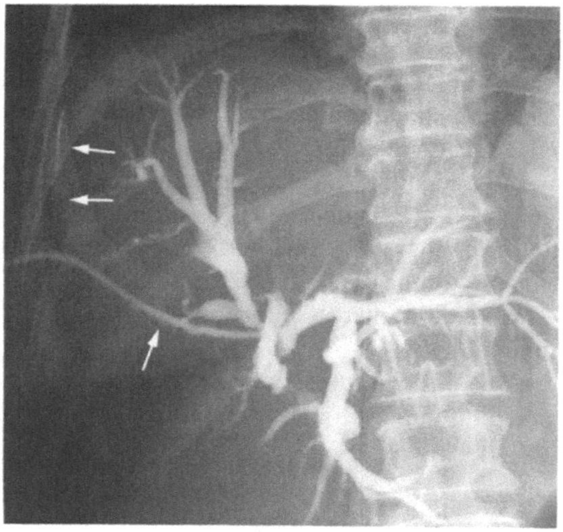

Fig. 45. Distal obstruction of the common bile duct due to a carcinoma of the head of the pancreas in a 67-year-old patient. External PTD: retrograde flow of contrast medium between catheter and drainage canal and opacification of a filiform fistula between liver and chest wall, indicating localised inflammation in the region of the drain tract

catheter width is 12-F) and a short course of antibiotics is given. Infections of the drainage canal can easily be recognised in the X-ray picture by the retrograde flow of contrast medium between catheter and parenchyma and the irregular limits of the drainage canal (Fig. 45).

In our experience, every catheter change is associated with a transitory inflammatory reaction in the biliary system, so that temporary antibiotic cover (orally, intravenously or directly through the catheter) should always be given. Like *Hoevels* et al. (1978), we regularly examine the bile draining from long-term indwelling drainage systems for micro-organisms, as the majority of these inflammations are clinically silent. Inflammation of the skin or chest wall can be avoided if the catheter is not stitched to the skin, but only affixed with strips of plaster.

10.3 Bile-Loss Syndrome

When bile is lost, bile acids and electrolytes (particularly sodium and bicarbonate) play a major role. The loss of bile acids results in disturbed fat and protein metabolism, which is easily recognised from the diarrhoea and fatty stools and can be picked up early by regular controls of the prothrombin time (Quick). As a rule, the patient cannot be expected to tolerate oral administration of the externally drained bile; instillation via nasogastric tubes over a long period of time is also only tolerable in emergency cases. It is recommended that the deficit in bile acids be compensated by substitution of the fat-soluble vitamins and programmed nutrition including fat from short-chain fatty acids (medium fatty triglyceride). It must, however be borne in mind that these have a low energy value, which must be compensated by an increased calorie intake. In addition, calcium should be substituted, as a disturbance in calcium absorption is associated with decreased fatty resorption. A special diet is not necessary, particularly as one is usually dealing with cancer patients who should be allowed a diet of choice, with additional substitution therapy depending on the clinical symptoms.

The patients lose electrolytes in bile, particularly sodium (up to 170 mEq/litre bile) and bicarbonate (up to 70 mEq/litre bile). Hyponatraemia may be manifested after a few days of drainage by the clinical symptoms of lethargy and personality changes. At the same time, metabolic acidosis may develop. Regular electrolyte checks should therefore be performed, with subsequent calculated substitution therapy.

None of our own three patients exhibited a bile-loss syndrome, as in every case some of the bile still managed to flow through the tight strictures into the small intestine.

10.4 Psychological Stress

An aspect of long-term indwelling PTD that has so far received little attention is the psychological disturbance experienced by the patient: despite the subjective feeling of well-being and possibly the complete integration into daily life, these patients are still constantly reminded of their incurable disease and are limited in their social relationships. The example of one of our own patients, who probably committed suicide, and similar observations obtained from larger centres, show that our task lies not only in technical management, but also in more intensive psychological guidance of patients with long-term PTD.

11 Comparison of PTD with Other Nonoperative Methods of Drainage and its Future

Besides PTD, various other methods of relieving biliary obstruction are currently in use.

11.1 Percutaneous Transhepatic Endoprostheses

Pereiras et al. (1977), *Burcharth* and *Nielbo* (1976), *Burcharth* et al. (1977), *Hoevels* et al. (1978, 1980a, 1980b), *Rupp* and *Weiss* (1980), *Hellekant* et al. (1980) and others have recently started to use percutaneously and transhepatically inserted endoprostheses more frequently than internal PTD. The main advantages claimed for this method are reduced psychological stress for the patient and a reduced incidence of cholangitis resulting from the drainage. For maintenance of the function of these endoprostheses it is evidently important that they have a certain minimum lumen and size and number of side-holes; *Rupp* and *Weiss* (1980) are so far the only authors who maintain that the endoprostheses allow more effective drainage than PTD, and attribute this to the wider lumen. On the other hand, the insertion of a

thicker endoprosthesis is only possible with a very rigid catheter and introducing wire system, which is associated with a higher rate of complications, mainly vascular (*Hoevels* et al. 1980a).
Burcharth and *Nielbo* (1976) published reports of fewer cases of cholangitis occurring with the use of endoprostheses than with internal PTD systems; the evaluation of this statement, however, presents problems, as most cases of cholangitis are not accompanied by clinical symptoms and only become overt on direct investigation of the bile, as *Hoevels* et al. (1978) have already reported. The conditions for possible reduction of the occurrence of cholangitis are (a) that the endoprosthesis is inserted immediately after PTC, and (b) that the distal end of the endoprosthesis lies in the common bile duct above the papilla.

Reports on the frequency of occlusions and dislocations of endoprostheses differ widely: *Hoevels* et al. (1980a) give an account of dysfunction caused by faulty insertion of the endoprosthesis in six of 13 cases; *Burcharth* et al. (1977) observed one instance of malposition and three of encrustation of the endoprosthesis amongst 41 cases, whilst *Pereiras* et al. (1977) did not find any dysfunction in their 12 patients.

On the basis of the higher complication rate, *Hoevels* et al. (1980a) consider the use of endoprostheses as indicated only in cases where adequate care of the PTD is not guaranteed or the PTD appears to cause the patient great psychological stress.

We regard internal PTD, with the option it allows of an external approach, preferable to the endoprosthesis, as it offers easy access from the outside whenever desired, should dysfunction or dislocation of the drain occur, which in the case of an endoprosthesis would always mean a renewed percutaneous transhepatic puncture and introduction of a new prosthesis. The risks of biliary tract infections can be kept very low by meticulous daily flushing, frequent catheter changes if required or covering of the external limb of the catheter with skin.

11.2 Transpapillary Endoprosthesis of the Pig-Tail Type

More recently, *Soehendra* (1980) has developed a method of inserting a 7-F pig-tail catheter 15 cm in length with side-holes into the common bile duct proximal to the stenosis by means of endoscopic guidance, using the transpapillary route after papillotomy. This method naturally demands great endoscopic skill. Compared with the percutaneously transhepatically inserted endoprosthesis, correction of a dysfunctioning or dislocated endoprosthesis is much simpler under these conditions.

11.3 Nasobiliary Tube

As a modification of the transpapillary endoprosthesis of the pig-tail type *Osnes* et al. (1979) and *Wurbs* (1980), working independently, developed a nasobiliary tube that is also inserted endoscopically. This tube drains to the outside via the intestinal tract and through the nose. *Wurbs* (1980) sees the greatest advantage in the possibility of the immediate access from the outside and the possibility of aspirating bile.

As yet there is insufficient experience to allow a good grasp of the difficulties, complication rates, and problems of the two methods just described. Whether the nasobiliary tube really is more tolerable for the patients than the PTD procedure can surely only be assessed in individual cases. External PTD has the advantage that the tubing and drainage bag can be hidden under the clothing, rather like a colostomy bag.

It is evident that the percutaneous transhepatically inserted endoprosthesis, the transpapillary endoprosthesis, and the nasobiliary tube can only be used in cases of tight stenosis in the hepatic bile ducts, and not where there is a complete tumour obstruction or in the presence of multiple obstructive sites in the region of the bifurcation of the hepatic bile duct. These methods should therefore be regarded as complementary to PTD.

As well as the diagnostic and therapeutic uses of PTD already described, there are many more extensions of this method which have not yet been adequately tried or tested:

- Cytological, bacteriological and biochemical examination of the bile can easily be carried out after aspiration from the catheter.
- Fine-needle biopsy or brush biopsies can be performed through the drainage catheter with no problem (*Mendez* et al. 1980).
- A transcatheteral fibre-cholangioscopy has as yet only been described by *Takada* et al. (1974) and has not found further use, probably for technical reasons. This method has rapidly gained importance since the introduction of intraductal radiotherapy by afterloading technique, as it offers a direct means of assessing the effect of the radiotherapy.
- Percutaneous antegrade papillotomy and splitting of stenoses have been described by *Günther* et al. (1982).
- The extent to which percutaneous infusion of cytostatic drugs into the biliary system represents a therapeutic alternative has not been adequately investigated.

12 Summary

In cases of obstructive jaundice percutaneous transhepatic cholangiography (PTC) together with endoscopic retrograde cholangiography (ERC) is the method of choice for the assessment operability and the most suitable operative procedure. Surprisingly, it has taken almost 35 years for percutaneous transhepatic biliary drainage to be developed from PTC and for it to be accepted in the treatment of obstructive jaundice. PTC itself now tends to be used as a preparation for biliary drainage rather than a method in the differential diagnosis of obstructive jaundice.

In a case of obstructive jaundice the indications for percutaneous transhepatic drainage (PTD) are as follows:

- Preoperative biliary decompression to reduce the high operative mortality associated with high serum bilirubin
- Palliative long-term biliary drainage in the case of inoperable malignancies
- Postoperative temporary splinting and drainage of a biliodigestive anastomosis to prevent anastomostic insufficiency
- Local therapy of acute suppurative cholangitis or liver abscess

Percutaneous transhepatic biliary drainage can be constructed as an externally draining system in the presence of a complete, biliary obstruction or, even better, as an internal system draining to the outside or internally into the duodenum in cases of very tight stenosis.

Our PTD technique differs fundamentally from that of other clinical workers:

1. The Swart special needle is used for the PTD. In contrast to the Chiba needle, this needle allows decongestion of the biliary system at the time of puncture, as well as the introduction of a guide wire into the biliary system, without reducing the accuracy of the puncture and without increasing the complication rate.
2. The puncture is performed in a diagonal craniocaudal direction, parallel to the course of the hepatic bile duct. This allows simpler insertion of the drainage catheter over the introducing wire into the biliary system, as the angle between the direction of puncture and the large central biliary ducts is small.
3. A Teflon tube is used to support the drainage catheter. This facilitates smooth introduction of a drainage catheter even if there is a tendency to kink between chest wall and liver or within the liver.

Experiences with 120 cases of PTD are reported; the problems and complications are discussed. The most common problem with this method is catheter displacement, which as a rule can easily be corrected without complications. Prevention consists of a careful choice of catheter and positioning. Despite CT and angiographic monitoring after PTD, we have not observed the alarming frequency of vascular complications described by other workers (*Tylén* et al. 1977; *Ueda* 1962). This type of complication is clearly reduced by our technique.

The advantages of PTD lie in the easy performance (after adequate experience) which, compared with a decompression operation, means less inconvenience and risk to the patient, the involvement of less technical equipment, and in the case of palliative indications a shorter period of hospitalisation.

PTD should influence the choice of surgical procedure in cases of obstructive jaundice, in that (a) patients with general or localised inoperability are spared a purely exploratory laparotomy, and (b) all operations purely for the purpose of biliary drainage in order to lower the high levels of serum bilirubin before a second operation should be replaced by PTD.

The improvement in the patients' general condition and operability after biliary decongestion is due to the recovery of liver parenchyma, the reduced bleeding tendency, and improvement in the hypoproteinaemic and nutritional state.

The combination of PTD with sequential hepatosplenic scintigraphy makes it possible, for the first time, to study the relationship between duration and extent of biliary obstruction and the development of a portal hypertension and also the reversibility of the portal hypertension after biliary drainage. Portal hypertension due to obstructive jaundice appears to be reversible after decongestion of the biliary tract. This provides a further explanation for the improved operability after biliary decompression.

Besides the decompression of the biliary system, PTD offers further therapeutic possibilities, such as dilatation of anastomotic strictures and gallstone crushing and extraction.

Patients with malignant obstructive jaundice after drainage can successfully be subjected to percutaneous localised radiotherapy via the indwelling PTD. To improve the radiotherapy, a technique of intraductal small space contact irradiation through the drainage canal has recently been developed which is more effective whilst sparing the surrounding healthy tissue, rather like gynaecological radiotherapy.

The combination of PTD and high-dose small-space irradiation promises an improvement in the palliative results that can be obtained in the treatment of malignant biliary obstructions, as well as a direct means of assessing the effect of radiotherapy on bile duct neoplasms by transcatheteral fibre-cholangioscopy.

Further developments can most certainly be expected in the diagnostic and therapeutic applications of the techniques described and those more recently developed, in addition to their use purely for biliary drainage.

References

Adolph K (1968) Gallengangs- und Pankreasdiagnostik. Enke, Stuttgart

Andrews WHH (1968) Functional difference between hepatic artery and portal vein regions. In: Brauer RW (ed) Liver function. American Institute of Biological Sciences, Washington

Anger HO (1958) Scintillation camera. Rev Sci Instr 29:27

Ariel JM, Pack GT (1960) The treatment of inoperable cancer of the biliary system with radioactive (131-J) rose bengal. J Roentgenol 83:474

Ariyama J, Shirakabe H, Ohashi K, Roberts GM (1978) Experience with percutaneous transhepatic cholangiography using the Japanese needle. Gastrointest Radiol 2:359

Atkinson MM, Happey MG, Smiddy FG (1960) New methods for diagnosis and research: percutaneous transhepatic cholangiography. Gut 1:357

Bear JW (1977) Hepatic arterioportal fistual related to a liver biopsy. Gastrointest Radiol 2:297

Bayindir S (1966) Percutane transhepatische Cholangiographie. ROFO 105:839

Bayindir S (1973) Percutane transhepatische Cholangiographie. In: Boecker W (ed) Gallenwege – Leber. Thieme, Stuttgart

Bedacht R, von Bary S (1975/76) Das Karzinom des Pankreas und Duodenums. Chir Praxis 20:379

Benjamin JS, Allison ME, Moule B, Blumgart LH (1978) The early use of fine-needle percutaneous transhepatic cholangiography in an approach to the diagnosis of jaundice in a surgical unit. Br J Surg 65:92

Biersack HJ (1978) Die Leberperfusion und ihre nicht-invasive Bestimmung anhand eines neu entwickelten Verfahrens. Habilitationsschrift, University of Bonn

Bilbao MK, Potter CT, Lee TG, Katon RM (1976) Complications of endoscopic retrograde cholangiography (ERCP): a study of 10,000 cases. Gastroenterology 70:314

Black HC, Hawk JC Jr, Rambo WM (1971) Long-term intubation of the biliary tract with silastic catheters. Am Surg 37:198

Blumgart LH (1976) Biliary tract obstruction: new approaches to old problems Am J Surg 135:19

Braasch JW, Gray BN (1977) Considerations that lower pancreatoduodenectomy mortality. Am J Surg 129:480

Brooks JR, Culebras JM (1976) Cancer of the pancreas. Palliative operation, Whipple procedure or total pancreatectomy? Am J Surg 131:516

Bünte H (1977) Therapie der Gallen- und Pankreastumoren. Monatskurse Aerztl Fortbild 27:410

Buckwalter HA, Lawton RL, Tidrick RT (1965) Bypass operations for neoplastic biliary obstructions. Am J Surg 109:100

Burcharth F, Nielbo N (1976) Percutaneous transhepatic cholangiography with selective catheterization of the common bile duct. AJR 127:409

Burcharth F, Jensen LJ, Olesen K (1977) Endoprosthesis for internal drainage of the biliary tract. Gastroenterology 77:133

Burckhardt H, Müller W (1921) Versuche über die Punktion der Gallenblase und ihre Röntgendarstellung. Dtsche Z Chir 162:168
Burhenne HJ (1972) Extraktion von Residualsteinen der Gallenwege ohne Reoperation. ROFO 117:425
Burhenne HJ (1974) The technique of biliary duct stones extraction; experience with 126 cases. Radiology 113:567
Burton-Opitz R (1911) Vascularity of the liver. II. The influence of the portal blood flow upon the flow in the hepatic artery. J Exp Physiol 4:93
Cahow CE (1979) Intrahepatic cholangiojejunostomy: a new simplified approach. Am J Surg 137:443
Carter FR, Saypol GM (1952) Transabdominal cholangiography. JAMA 148:148
Catell RB, Pyrtek LJ (1949) An appraisal of pancreatoduodenal resection. Ann Surg 129:840
Classen H, Wenz W, von Fritsch E (1973) Pankreasdarstellung. Kombination von retrograder Pankreaticographie und Coeliacographie. Dtsch Med Wochenschr 98:1524
Committee for Radiation Oncology Studies (1976) Radiation therapy and surgery. Cancer 37:2084
Corlette MB, Bookwalter JR (1980) Individualisation of treatment for hilar bile duct cancers. Cancer 46:415
Coutsoftides T, McDonald J, Shibata HR (1977) Carcinoma of the pancreas and periampullary region: a 41-year experience. Ann Surg 186:730
Crile G (1970) The advantages of bypass operation over radical pancreatoduodenectomy in the treatment of pancreatic carcinoma. Surg Gynecol Obstet 130:1049
Cynn WS, Levin BL, Gureghian PA, Chait A (1979) Infusion hepatotomography for evaluation of obstructive jaundice. AJR 132:187
Dammermann R, Zilly W, Trübzsch D, Lindner H, Kirchhoff M (1978) Die Bedeutung der perkutanen transhepatischen Cholangiographie (PTC) mit ultradünner Nadel in der Differentialdiagnose der Cholestase. Dtsch Med Wochenschr 103:371
Dawson JL (1965) Post-operative renal function in obstructive jaundice: effects of mannitol diuresis. Br Med J 1:82
Dick W, Dortemann J (1965) Die Behandlung hochsitzender maligner Gallengangsstenosen. Langenbecks Arch Klin Chir 311:83
Dittel KK, Kraft E, Trömer W (1978) Der heutige Stand der Gallenchirurgie. Z Allg Med 54:206
Dobelbower RP, Borgelt BB, Strubler KA, Kutcher GJ, Suntharalingam N (1980) Precision radiotherapy for cancer of the pancreas: technique and results. Int J Radiat Oncol Biol Phys 6:1127
Dotter CT (1980) Transluminal angioplasty: a long review. Radiology 135:561
Elias HE, Sherrick JC (1969) Morphology of the liver. Academic, New York
Emrich D (1979) Nuklearmedizin. Funktionsdiagnostik und Therapie. Thieme, Stuttgart
Enderling F (1974) Karzinome der Gallenblase und des Hauptgallenganges. Helv Chir Acta 41:705
Evans JA (1973) In: Margulis AR, Burhenne HJ (eds) Alimentary tract roentgenology, vol 2. Mosby St. Louis, p 1339
Feduska NJ, Deut TL, Lindenauer SM (1971) Results of palliative operations for carcinoma of the pancreas. Arch Surg 103:330
Felci L, Felci V (1957) Colangiografia transhepatica percutanea. Radiol Med (Torino) 43:591
Ferruci JT, Mueller PR, Harbin WP (1980) Percutaneous transhepatic biliary drainage. Radiology 135:1
Fischer A, Takacs L (1964) Über die Regulation des Kreislaufs in der Leber. Acta Physiol Acad Sci Hung 24:433
Flemma RJ, Schauble JF, Gardner CE, Anlyan WG, Capp MP (1963) Percutaneous transhepatic cholangiography in the differential diagnosis of jaundice. Surg Gynecol Obstet 116:556
Fletcher MS, Brinkley D, Dawson JL, Nunnerley H, Wheeler PG, Williams R (1981) Treatment of high bileduct carcinoma by internal radiotherapy with Iridium-192 wire. Lancet 25:172
Fortner JG, Kim DK, Cubilla A, Turnbull A, Pahnke LD, Shils ME (1977) Regional pancreatectomy: en bloc pancreatic, portal vein and lymph node resection. Ann Surg 186:42

Friedland HM (1971) Leiomyosarcoma of the gallbladder. J Med Soc NJ 68:205
Funck-Brentano JL, Mery JP, Vantelon J, Watchi J (1963) Les insuffisances rénales aiguës de l'angiocholite urémique (18 observations personelles). Presse Med 71:1039
Glenn F, Thorbjanarson B (1964) Carcinoma of the pancreas. Ann Surg 159:945
Göthlin J, Transberg KG (1973) Complications of percutaneous transhepatic cholangiography (PTC) AJR 117:426
Goetze O (1951) Die transhepatische Dauerdrainage bei der hohen Gallengangsstenose. Langenbecks Arch Klin Chir 270:97
Goldberg HJ, Filly RA, Korobkin M, Moss AA, Kressel HY, Callen PW (1978) Capability of CT body scanning and ultrasound to demonstrate the status of the biliary ductal system in patients with jaundice. Radiology 129:731
Green N, Mikkelsen WP, Kernen JA (1973) Cancer of the common hepatic bile ducts – palliative radiotherapy. Radiology 109:687
Gudjonsson B, Livstone EM, Spiro HM (1978) Cancer of the pancreas. Diagnostic accuracy and survival statistics. Cancer 42:2494
Günther R, Rückert K, Mangold G (1979) Perkutane Gallenwegsdrainage in Feinnadelpunktionstechnik. Dtsch Med Wochenschr 104:51
Günther R, Georgi M, Schaeffer HJ (1980) Transvenöse Cholangiographie und perkutane transhepatische Feinnadelcholangiographie. Dtsch Med Wochenschr 105:255
Günther R, Klose K, Schmidt HD (1982) Perkutane Gallenwegsdrainage und therapeutische Kathetereingriffe. Paper given at Deutscher Röntgenkongreß 1982, Berlin
Hanafee WN, Weiner M (1967) Transjugular percutaneous cholangiography. Radiology 88:35
Hanna SS, Rider WD (1978) Carcinoma of the gallbladder or extrahepatic bile ducts: the role of radiotherapy. Can Med Assoc 118:59
Hannsson JA, Hoevels J, Simert G, Tylén U, Vang J (1979) Clinical aspects of nonsurgical percutaneous transhepatic bile drainage in obstructive lesions of the extrahepatic bile ducts. Ann Surg 189:58
Hanson KM, Johnson PC (1963) Hepatic artery pressure – flow relationships in the in situ dog liver. Physiologist 6:197
Hanson KM, Johnson PC (1966) Local control of hepatic arterial and portal venous blood flow in the dog. J Physiol 211:712
Harbin WP, Ferucci JT Jr (1980) Nonoperative management of malignant biliary obstruction: A radiologic alternative. AJR 135:103
Harbin WP, Mueller PR, Ferrucci JT (1980) Transhepatic cholangiography: complications and use patterns of the fine-needle technique. Radiology 135:15
Hartenbach W (1977) Erfahrungsbericht über die Anwendung einer Gallengangs-Endoprothese. Chirurg 48:549
Hashmonai M, Lev L, Schramek A, Ben-Arieh Y, Robinson E (1980) Long survival following combined treatment of inoperable cholangiocarcinoma: surgery, radiotherapy and chemotherapy. J Surg Oncol 13:231
Havrilla TR, Haaga JR, Alfidi RJ, Reich NE (1977) Computed tomography and obstructive biliary disease. Am J Roentgenol 128:765
Hawkins JF Jr, McNeely GF, Weaver DL Jr (1976) Percutaneous antecubital transvenous cholangiography. A modified technique using a flexible needle. Radiology 120:423
Heim W, Cramer W (1960) Über Gallengangsanastomosen. Chirurg 31:248
Hellekant C (1976) Vascular complications following needle puncture of the liver. Acta Radiol [Diagn] (Stockh) 17:202
Hellekant C, Jonsson K, Genell S (1980) Percutaneous internal drainage in obstructive jaundice. AJR 134:661
Hermann AH, Egdahl RH, Williams LF, Wittenburg J, Nabseth DC (1974) Problems engered by a 'standard approach' to the patients with jaundice or biliary pain. J Surg 127:404
Herskovic A, Heaston D, Engler MJ, Fishburn RJ, Jones RS, Noell KT (1981) Irradiation of biliary carcinoma. Radiology 139:219
Hertzberg J (1974) Pancreatico-duodenal resection and by-pass operation in patients with carcinoma of the head of the pancreas, ampulla and distal end of the common duct. Acta Chir Scand 140:523
Hess W (1965) Surgery of the biliary passages and the pancreas. Van Nostrand, New York, p 474

Hess W (1977) Nachoperationen an den Gallenwegen. Enke, Stuttgart
Heydenrych JJ, du T van Zijl FD, van Zyl JJW (1969) Surg Oncol 1:63
Hines C, Ferrante WA, Davis WD (1972) Percutaneous transhepatic cholangiography experience with 102 procedures. Am J Dig Dis 17:868
Hoevels J, Lunderquist A, Ihse I (1978) Percutaneous transhepatic intubation of bile ducts for combined internal–external drainage in preoperative and palliative treatment of obstructive jaundice. Gastrointest Radiol 3:28
Hoevels J, Nilsson U (1980a) Intrahepatic vascular lesion following nonsurgical percutaneous transhepatic bile duct intubation. Gastrointest Radiol 5:127
Hoevels J, Lunderquist A, Owmann T, Ihse I (1980b) A large-bore Teflon endoprosthesis with side-holes for nonoperative decompression of the biliary tract in malignant obstructive jaundice. Gastrointest Radiol 5:361
Huard P, Do-Xuan-Hop (1937) La ponction transhépatic des canaux biliares. Bull Soc Med Chir Indochine 15:1090
Hudgins PT, Meoz RT (to be published) Radiation therapy for obstructive jaundice secondary to tumor malignancy. Int J Radiat Oncol Biol Phys
Ihse I, Lilja P, Arnesjö B, Bengmark S (1977) Total pancreatectomy for cancer. An appraisal of 65 cases. Ann Surg 186:675
Irish CB, Meaney TF (1980) Percutaneous transhepatic cholangiography. AJR 134:137
Isley JK, Schauble JF Jr (1962) Interpretation of the percutaneous transhepatic cholangiography. Am J Roentgenol 88:772
Iwasaki V, Ohto M, Todoroki T, Okamwa T, Nishimura A, Sato H (1977) Treatment of carcinoma of the biliary system. Surg Gynecol Obstet 144:219
Kadell BM, Weiner M (1973) Current status of the transjugular approach for direct cholangiography. Surg Clin North Am 53:1019
Katon RM, Lee TG, Parent JA, Bilbao MK, Smith FW (1974) Endoscopic retrograde cholangiography (ERCP): experience with 100 cases. Am J Dig Dis 19:295
Keighley MRB (1977) Micro-organisms in the bile. A preventable cause of sepsis after biliary surgery. Ann R Coll Surg Engl 59:328
Keighley MRB, Lister DM, Jacobs SI (1974) Hazards of surgical treatment due to microorganisms in the bile. Surgery 75:578
Kennedy AC, Burton JA, Luke RG, Briggs JD, Lindsay RM, Allison MEM, Edward N, Dargie HJ (1973) Factors affecting prognosis in acute renal failure. QJ Med 42:73
Kidd HA (1950) Percutaneous transhepatic cholangiography. Arch Surg 72:262
Kim WS, Barth KH, Zinner M (1982) Seeding of pancreatic carcinoma along the transhepatic catheter tract. Radiology 143:427
Köster R, Swart B, Terwort H (1979) Perkutane transhepatische Gallengangsdrainage zur praeoperativen und palliativen Behandlung der Gallengangsobstruktion. Radiologe 19:394
Kopelson G, Harisiadis L, Tretter P, Chang CH (1977) The role of radiation therapy in cancer of the extrahepatic biliary system. Int J Radiat Oncol Biol Phys 2:883
Krain LS (1972) Gallbladder and extra-hepatic bile duct carcinoma. Geriatrics 27:111
Kremer K, Berghaus H, Düwell J, Filthaut W (1967) Erfolgsaussichten von Radikaleingriffen bei den sog. periampullären Karzinomen. Chirurg 38:278
Lam CR (1940) The present status of carcinoma of the gallbladder: a study of thirty-four cases. Ann Surg 111:403
Lee WJ (1942) Evaluation of peritoneoscopy in intraabdominal diagnosis. Rev Gastroenterol 9:133
Leger L, Zara M, Arvay N (1952) Cholangiographie et drainage biliaire par ponction transhépatique. Presse Med 60:936
Levitt RG, Sagel SS, Stanley RJ, Jost RG (1977) Accuracy of computed tomography of the liver and biliary tract. Radiology 124:123
Luska G, Elgeti H, Wanner K, Rumpf KD, Gerber R (1981) Computertomographie (CT) beim tumorbedingten Verschlußikterus zur Therapieplanung und zur Planung der perkutanen transhepatischen Gallenwegsdrainage (PTCD). ROFO 134:28
Maki T, Sato T, Kakizaki G (1966) Pancreatoduodenectomy for periampullary carcinomas. Arch Surg 92:825
Mendez G, Russell E, Levi JU, Koolpe H, Cohen M (1980) Percutaneous brush biopsy and internal drainage of biliary tree through endoprosthesis. AJR 134:653

Moertel GC (1973) Extrahepatic bile ducts. In: Holland JF, Frei E (eds) Cancer medicine, Sect 24, Chap 5. Lea & Febiger, Philadelphia, p 1555
Molnar W, Stockum A (1974) Relief of obstructive jaundice through percutaneous transhepatic catheter – a new therapeutic method. AJR 122:356
Molnar W, Stockum A (1978) Transhepatic dilatation of choledochoenterostomy strictures. Radiology 129:59
Mongé JJ, Judd ES, Gagl RP (1964) Radical pancreatoduodenectomy: a 22-year experience with the complications, mortality rate and survival rate. Ann Surg 160:711
Moossa AR, Anagnost M, Hall AW, Moraldi A, Skinner DB (1975) The continuing challenge of gallbladder cancer. Am J Surg 130:57
Mori K, Mirumi A, Sugiyama M, Okabe M, Matsucka T, Ishii J, Masanobu A (1977) Percutaneous transhepatic bile drainage. Ann Surg 185:111
Morris AI, Faurcitt RA, Wood R, Forbes WSC, Isherwood I, Marsh MN (1977) Computed tomography in the diagnosis of disorders of excessive iron storage of the liver. J Comput Assist Tomogr 1:101
Nakase A, Matsumato Y, Uchida K, Honjo I (1977) Surgical treatment of cancer of the pancreas and the periampullary region: cumulative results in 57 institutions in Japan. Ann Surg 185:52
Nakayama T, Ikeda A, Okuda K (1978) Percutaneous transhepatic drainage of the biliary tract. Gastroenterology 74:554
Nebel OT, Formes MF (1973) Endoscopic pancreato-cholangiography. Ann J Dig Dis 18:1042
Nettelblad SC (1954) Die Lobierung und innere Topographie der Säuglingsleber. Acta Nat (Basel) [Suppl] 20:1954
Neugebauer W, Durst J, Mayer HR (1979) Das primäre Carcinom der extrahepatischen Gallenwege. Langenbecks Arch Chir 350:33
Nurick AW, Patey DH, Whiteside CG (1953) Percutaneous transhepatic cholangiography in the diagnosis of obstructive jaundice. Br J Surg 41:27
Okuda K, Tanikawa K, Emura T, Kuratomi S, Jinnouchi S, Urabe K, Sumikoshi T, Kanda Y, Fukuyama Y, Musha H, Mori H, Shimokawa Y, Yakushiji F, Matsuura Y (1974) Nonsurgical percutaneous transhepatic cholangiography – diagnostic significance in medical problems of the liver. Dig Dis 19:1
Okuda K, Musha H, Nakajiama Y, Takayasu K, Suzuki Y, Morita M, Yamasaki T (1978) Frequency of intrahepatic arteriovenous fistula as a sequela to percutaneous needle puncture of the liver. Gastroenterology 74:1204
Oldendorf WH, Kitano M, Shimizu S (1965) Evaluation of a simple technique for abrupt intravenous injection of radioisotope. J Nucl Med 6:205
Oleaga JA, Ring EJ, Freiman DB, McLean GK, Rosen RJ (1980) Extension of neoplasm along the tract of a transhepatic tube. AJR 135:841
Olsson O, Tylén U (1972) Angiography in carcinoma at the papilla of Vater (1971). Acta Radiol (Stockh) 12:375
Osnes M, Geiran O, Grönoeth K, Havig Ø (1979) Nonoperative internal drainage of obstructive common bile ducts. Arch Surg 114:862
Otho M, Ohno T, Tsuchiya V, Saisho H (1973) Percutaneous transhepatic cholangiography. Igakushoin, Tokyo
Ozdemir AJ, Lancaster JR (1971) Percutaneous transhepatic cholangiography. Arch Surg 103:684
Peabody CN, Millmann M (1972) Vitallium tube repair of a bile duct stricture. A quarter century survivor. J Surg 124:413
Peiper HJ, Kallenberg A, Giersberg O (1967) Die perkutane transhepatische Cholangiographie. Langenbecks Arch Klin Chir 317:232
Pereiras R, Hudson D, Viamonte M, Mejia J, Schiff E (1977) Percutaneous transhepatic insertion of a permanent biliary tract prothesis. A new non-surgical method for the relief of obstructive jaundice. Presented at the Scientific Assembly and Annual Meeting of the Radiological Society of North America, Chicago
Pipelich MV, Lambert PM (1978) Radiotherapy of carcinomas of the extrahepatic biliary system. Radiology 127:767
Popper H, Jefferson NC, Necheles N (1954) Survival of dogs after partial or total devascularization of the liver. Ann Surg 140:93

Popper H, Schaffner F (1957) Liver: Structure and function. Mc Graw-Hill, New York
Priestley JT, Wollaeger EE (1961) Malignant lesions of the bile ducts and head of the pancreas. Surg Clin North Am 41:963
Prioton JB (1960) La ponction extrapéritonéale du foie, son intérêt pour la biopsie hépatique et la cholangiographie percutanée. Presented at the 1st meeting of the Societé de Médecine Biologique, Montpellier, 1st April 1968
Rappaport AM (1960) Betrachtungen zur Pathophysiologie der Leberstruktur. Klin Wochenschr 38:561
Reichart W, Ihse J (1980) Percutaneous transhepatic portography in pancreatic carcinoma. Diagnosis and evaluation of resectability. Acta Radiol [Diagn] (Stockh) 21:579
Remolar J, Katz S, Rybak B, Pellizari O (1956) Percutaneous transhepatic cholangiography. Gastroenterology 31:39
Rettenmaier G (1977) Ultraschalluntersuchung beim Cholestasesyndrom. Presented at the 3rd Bremer Gastroenterologisches Symposium, Bremen 8. 10. 1977
Reuter RS, Chuang VP (1976) The location of increased resistance to portal blood flow in obstructive jaundice. Invest Radiol 11:54
Ring EJ, Oleaga J, Freiman D, Husted J, Lunderquist A (1978) Therapeutic applications of catheter cholangiography. Radiology 128:333
Ring EJ, Husted JW, Oleaga JA (1979) A multihole catheter for maintaining longterm percutaneous antegrade biliary drainage. Radiology 132:752
Rösch J, Antonovic R, Dotter CT (1975) Transjugular approach to the liver, biliary system and portal circulation. J Roentgenol 125:602
Ross DE (1959) Cancer of the pancreas. Am J Gastroenterol 31:517
Roux P, Larimore LD (1920) The biliary factor in liver lesions. J Exp Med 32:249
Royer M, Solari AV, Lottery-Canari R (1942) La cholangiografia noquirurgica: nuevo metode exploracion de las vias biliares. Arch Argent Dig Nutr 17:368
Rückert K, Günther R, Kümmerle F (1979) Praeoperative perkutane transhepatische Gallenwegsdrainage (PTCD) beim malignen Verschlußikterus. Langenbecks Arch chir 349:556
Rupp N, Weiss H-D (1980) Perkutan eingebrachte Gallengangsprothesen als Primärmaßnahme bei Verschlußikterus. ROFO 133:279
Rüttimann A, Wellauer J, Schamann M, Akovbiantz A, Middendorp U (1965) Die perkutane transhepatische Cholangiographie. Schweiz Med Wochenschr 95:124
Santos M, Figuerva L, Lopez O (1960) Percutaneous transhepatic cholangiography in the diagnosis of posthepatic jaundice. Surgery 48:295
Sato T, Saitoh Y, Koyama K, Watanabe K (1968) Preoperative determination of operability in carcinomas of the pancreas and the periampullary region. Ann Surg 168:876
Sauerwein K (1976) Tumornahbestrahlungsgerät zur interstitiellen und intracavitären Anwendung mit vorwählbarem Isodosenprogramm. Med Phys 2:453
Scherer U, Lissner J, Brall B, Eisenburg J, Zrenner M, Schildberg F-W (1979) Computertomographie der Leber. ROFO 130:531
Schmidt HD, Rückert R, Brunner H (1977) Der maligne Verschlußikterus. Gastroenterol 15:89
Schütt H, Köster R (1979) Technik und diagnostische Wertigkeit der perkutanen transhepatischen Cholangiographie. Roentgenblätter 32:491
Schwiegk H (1932) Untersuchungen über die Leberdurchblutung und den Pfortaderkreislauf. Naunyn/Schmiedebergs Arch Exp Pathol Pharmacol 168:693
Shaldon S, Barber KM, Young WB (1962) Percutaneous transhepatic cholangiography. Gastroenterology 42:371
Shamiyeh F (1974) Das primäre Gallenblasencarcinom. Dtsch Med Wochenschr 99:1583
Shapiro TM (1975) Adenocarcinoma of the pancreas: a statistical analysis of biliary bypass vs. Whipple resection in good risk patients. Ann Surg 182:715
Sivaprasad R, Gopalaswamy N (1980) Jaundice: an internists perspective. Radiol Clin North Am 18:179
Smith HW, Engel C, Averbrook B, Longmire WP Jr (1969) Problems of retained and recurrent common bile duct stones. Surgery 66:291
Smith R (1964) Hepaticojejunostomy–choledochojejunostomy, a method of intrajejunal anastomosis. Br J Surg 51:183
Smoron GL (1977) Radiation therapy of carcinoma of gallbladder and biliary tract. Cancer 40:1422

Soehendra N (1980) Transpapilläre Endoprothesen vom pig-tail-Typ. Technik, Instrumentarium, Risiko, Resultate. Presented at the 11th International Congress of Gastroenterology, Hamburg, June 1980
Spieler U, Largiadér F, Amman R (1977) Diagnose and Therapie von Stenosen oder Verschlüssen der intrahepatischen Gallenwege. Helv Chir Acta 44:471
Suzuki T, Manabe T, Tani T, Tobe T (1980) Angiography and pancreatoductography in resectable carcinoma of the pancreas. Acta Radiol [Diagn] (Stockh) 21:587
Swart B (1968) Die perkutane transhepatische Cholangiographie. In: Bartelheimer H, Heisig N (eds) Aktuelle Gastroenterologie. Thieme, Stuttgart
Swart B, Meyer G, Hermann FJ (1976) Röntgendiagnostik der Gallenblase und Gallenwege. In: Handbuch der medizinischen Radiologie, vol XII/1. Springer, Berlin Heidelberg New York, p 305
Schenk WG, Menno AD, Murray NA, Drapanas T (1960) Applications of the electromagnetic flowmeter to vascular studies in human patients. Surgery 48:221
Stanley RJ, Sagel SS, Levitt RG (1977) Computed tomography of the liver. Radiol Clin North Am 15:331
Stern RB, Knill Jones RP, Williams R (1973) Pitfalls in the diagnosis of jaundice due to carcinoma of the pancreas or biliary tree. Br Med J 1:533
Strunk E, Clemens M, Langhans P (1979) Chirurgische Therapie bei malignem Verschlußikterus. Leber Magen Darm 9:192
Tabrisky J, Lindstrom RL, Hamelin LG, Pfisterer WF (1976) Chiba percutaneous transhepatic cholangiography. A valuable method for visualizing the nondilated biliary tract. Am J Roentgenol 126:755
Takada T, Suzuki S, Nakamura M (1974) Percutaneous cholangioscopy. Gastrointest Endosc 16:106
Takada T, Hanyu F, Kobayashi S, Uchida Y (1976) Percutaneous transhepatic cholangial drainage: direct approach under fluoroscopic control. J Surg Oncol 8:83
Teisseive R, Marty MH, Clanet J, Fourtainier G, Putois J (1978) L'abord hépatique par voie transjugulaire dans le diagnostic des ictères et l'exploration du système porte. J Radiol Electrol 59:531
Terblanche J, Lower JH (1973) U-Tube drainage in the palliative therapy of carcinoma of the main hepatic duct junction. Surg Clin North Am 53:1245
Terblanche J, Saunders SJ, Lower JH (1972) Prolonged palliation in carcinoma of the main hepatic duct junction. Surgery 71:720
Thelen M, Paquet KJ, Schulz D, Herpertz C (1977) Ergebnisse der transjugulären antegraden Cholangio- und retrograden Cholangio- und retrograden Portographie. Roentgenblätter 30:508
Todoroki T, Tsunemoto H, Iwasaki Y, Usui S (1976) Radiological effects of single massive irradiation on the liver hilum of rabbits. Jp J Gastroenterol Surg 9:474
Treadwell TA, Hardin WJ (1976) Primary carcinoma of the gallbladder. Am J Surg 132:703
Tylén U, Hoevels J, Vang J (1977) Percutaneous transhepatic cholangiography with external drainage of obstructive biliary lesions. Surg Gynecol Obstet 144:13
Ueda H (1962) Circulation of hepatic artery and portal vein. In: Martini GA (ed) Aktuelle Probleme der Hepatologie. Thieme, Stuttgart
Ukai T, Ohshima S, Kuriyama H, Asoh R, Okamura J, Murakami F (1971) A new device for external biliary drainage using percutaneous transhepatic cholangiography. Med J Osaka Univ 22:85
Van Heerden JA, Judd ES, Dockerty MB (1967) Carcinoma of the extra-hepatic bile ducts. Am J Surg 113:49
Vaittenen E (1970) Carcinoma of the gallbladder: a study of 390 cases diagnosed in Finland 1953–1967. Ann Chir Gynaecol Fenn [Suppl] 168:1
Walters W, Olson PF (1935) Papillary colloid adenocarcinoma of the extra-hepatic bile ducts. Minn Med 18:460
Wannagat L (1973) Laparoskopische Cholangiographie. Radiologe 13:26
Wannagat L (1974) Laparoskopische Cholecystographie und transhepatische Cholangiographie. In: Demling L (ed) Klinische Gastroenterologie, vol II. Thieme, Stuttgart, p 887

Warren KW, Catell RB, Blackburn JP, Nora PF (1962) A long term appraisal of pancreaticoduodenal resection for peri-ampullary carcinoma. Ann Surg 155:653
Wenz W (1967) Angiographische Darstellung der Gallenblasenarterien. ROFO 106:381
Williams RD, Elliot DW, Zollinger RW (1960) The effect of hypotension in obstructive jaundice. Arch Surg. 81:335
Wurbs D (1980) Nasobiliäre Sonde. Technik, Belästigung, Risiko. Presented at the 11th International Congress of Gastroenterology, Hamburg, June 1980
Zeitler E, Grüntzig A, Schoop W (eds) (1978) Percutaneous vascular recanalization. Springer, Berlin Heidelberg New York
Zinberg SS, Berk JE, Plasencia H (1965) Percutaneous transhepatic cholangiography: its use and limitations. Am J Dig Dis 10:154
Zoeckler CE (1975) Hämodynamik der portalen Hypertension. In: Zoeckler CE, Georghiu T (eds) Die portale Hypertension. Witzstrock, Baden-Baden

Videodensitometric Measurements of the Blood Flow in the Model Circulation and in the Iliac Arteries: Methodological Investigations

H. Fröhlich [1]

1 From the Department of Radiology, University of Hannover Medical School, Hannover, West Germany (Direktor: Prof. Dr. H. St. Stender).
Present address: Röntgenabteilung des Robert-Koch-Krankenhauses, von Rhedenstraße 1, D-3011 Gehrden. Submitted for publication in September 1983

1 Introduction

The quantitative analysis of blood flow within central and peripheral blood vessels has attracted more and more interest, for with the rapid developments in vascular surgery and the introduction of percutaneous transluminal angioplasty, it is becoming increasingly important to be able to measure regional blood flow in man. In clinical radiology, angiography has been used predominantly from the point of view of its morphological applications. However, theoretically angiography may also be regarded as a specific application of indicator-dilution measurements of blood flow. The indicator is contrast medium (CM), the changing concentration of which is recorded by cinematography or video-electronic systems at sites downstream from the point of injection. The curves of density thus obtained correspond to indicator-dilution curves. The blood flow can be calculated from the concentration-time curves of CM in much the same way as it is estimated from other indicator-dilution curves.

In our early work with clinical application of videodensitometric measurement of blood flow in the iliac artery, we found that this method did not offer as high a degree of accuracy as one would have expected from investigations by other authors. We saw that we needed to examine the following problems:

1. We had to investigate whether our conventional X-ray equipment and videodensitometer could be viewed as a linear measuring system. To what extent do unavoidable nonlinear changes in the measuring signals influence the blood flow values?
2. From our initial investigations we had gained the impression that the oscillating nature of the blood flow has an influence on the reproducibility and accuracy of the measurements. This problem needed to be investigated further.
3. Lastly, in our opinion the extensive analysis required to interpret density curves is an important factor in discouraging more widespread clinical application of densitometric blood flow measurements.

1.1 Basic Concept of Videodensitometric Blood Flow Measurements

The X-rays from the X-ray tube permeate the object under investigation and are intensified electronically through an image intensifier. The light image on the output screen of the intensifier is scanned by a television camera and its output voltage is fed into a videodensitometer. Two electronic sampling windows in the videodensitometer register from the video image the voltage which results from the X-ray absorption caused by an injected CM bolus. Therefore the densitometer output voltage is equivalent to an indicator mass curve.

One method of densitometric flow measurement in a blood vessel is based upon the determination of transit time of CM between two measuring points. If Δl is the distance between the measuring points and Δt is the transit time of a CM bolus the blood flow can be calculated by the following formula:

$$F = \frac{\Delta l}{\Delta t} \cdot \pi \cdot \frac{d^2}{4} \qquad (1)$$

where d is the diameter of the vessel (Fig. 1).

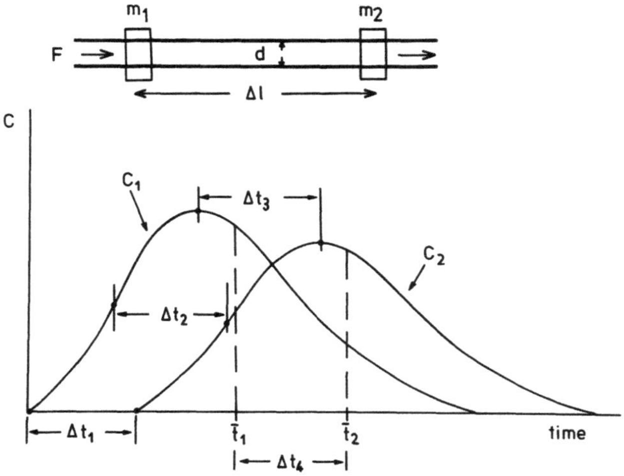

Fig. 1. *Upper panel:* Principle of flow measurement in blood vessels with two densitometric sampling windows m_1 and m_2. *Lower panel:* several methods to determine the transit time (Δt) of two densitometer curves (C_1 and C_2). Δt_1, time between the points of the first arrival; Δt_2, time between the points of half-maximum; Δt_3, time between the maxima of amplitude; Δt_4, time between the lines of gravity (i.e. mean time $\bar{t}_2$ of the curves C_1 and C_2)

Several methods have been suggested for the determination of the transit time Δt. The transit time is the difference between the arrival times at corresponding points of the two indicator mass curves, i.e. the points of first arrival, the points of half-maximum and maximum amplitude, and the points of mean time (Fig. 1).

The first three points are often not precisely determinable from the curves, or reflect only the faster moving particles of the radiopaque indicator at the front of the bolus. It is also assumed that the CM bolus does not change in shape as it passes between the two measuring points. Conventionally, therefore, the mean time, that is the line of gravity of the density curves, has been accepted as the point used for determination of the transit time, since all particles of the radiopaque indicator are taken into account (*Rutishauser* 1969).

The mean transit time is represented by the formula:

$$\Delta t = \bar{t}_2 - \bar{t}_1 = \frac{\int_0^\infty C_2 \cdot (t) \cdot t \cdot dt}{\int_0^\infty C_2 \cdot (t) \cdot dt} - \frac{\int_0^\infty C_1 \cdot (t) \cdot t \cdot dt}{\int_0^\infty C_1 \cdot (t) \cdot dt} \qquad (2)$$

where C_1 and C_2 are the concentrations of the CM of the two densitometer curves. This method of calculation will be called the line-of-gravity method.

A rather different mathematical approach for calculation of the transit time is the cross-correlation function ($F_{1,2}$) of the two densitometer curves (C_1, C_2) according to the mathematical relationship:

$$F_{1,2}(\tau) = \frac{1}{T_0} \cdot \int_0^\infty C_1(t-\tau)\, C_2(t)\, dt \qquad (3)$$

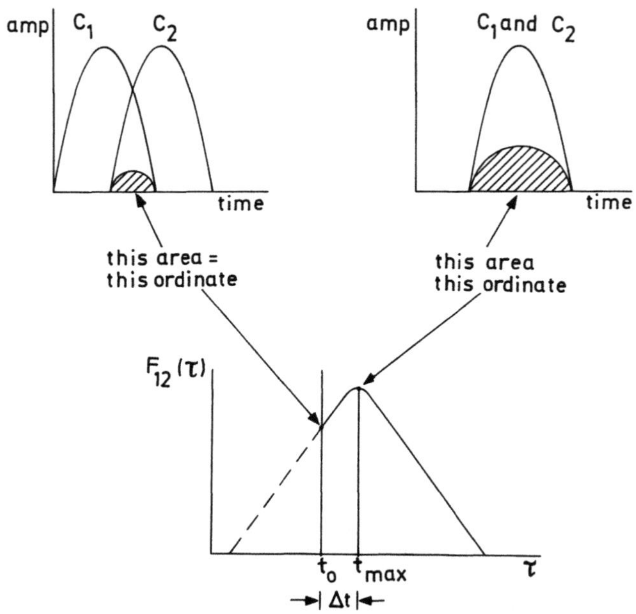

Fig. 2. Graphic interpretation of the cross-correlation function [$F_{1,2}$ (τ)]. Signal C_2 is fixed while signal C_1 is shifted in time over it until the two signals have a maximum overlap. The time Δt between the start of the shifting (t_0) and the overlap (t_{max}) is the desired transit time. (Modified after Rosen and Silverman)

The correlation works on the principle of templated matching (*Rosen* and *Silverman* 1973). One of the signals is fixed, the other one is electronically shifted in time over the stationary one until there is maximum overlap, i.e. until a match is obtained. The time of signal shifting to get the overlap corresponds to the bolus transit time. A graphic interpretation of cross-correlation is given in Fig. 2.

2 Calibrating the Roentgen-Video Equipment

2.1 Introduction

The linear course of the transfer function of an X-ray–television chain used as measuring system is dependent on several physical factors. The radiation emitted from the X-ray tube passes through an absorbing medium and is attenuated by photoabsorption and by the Compton scattering effect according to the Lambert-Beer law; after adequate filtering one can achieve quasi-monochromatic radiation. The radiation which has passed through the absorbing medium is converted into a light image on the input screen of an image intensifier tube. Photoelectric optics intensify the input image into a considerably lighter output image, which is fed by an optical system onto the photoelectric layer of a television camera.

If one considers the fluoroscopic equipment outlined above as a tool for measuring the density of an object, then a transfer function emerges, in that the linear density variation in an object is reproduced by exponential variation in the video voltage. Therefore the video voltage is converted to a logarithm before integration, so that the densitometer output voltage responds linearly to linear changes in the density of the object.

The validity of the Lambert-Beer law for radiodensitometry as a function of the wavelength of radiation as well as the concentration and thickness of CM has been proven by several authors (*Bürsch* et al. 1969; *Lantz* and *Strid* 1973; *Rutishauser* 1969). Therefore, in recording the overall transfer function of our X-ray–television chain, we confined ourselves entirely to the measurement conditions of our clinical investigation, as follows:

1. The roentgen tube voltage and the radiation filtration were chosen in such a way that the signal-to-noise ratio in the television image still allowed a sufficiently accurate view of details.
2. The opening of the lead diaphragm was adjusted in such a way that the fluoroscopic image had the size required to show a longer vessel segment.
3. The thickness of the CM stepwedge corresponded to the diameter of a large iliac artery.
4. The unavoidable effect of radiation scattering in the patient upon the overall transfer function was compensated by inserting a 13-cm-thick layer of water in the radiation field.

2.2 Method and Materials

We used a plexiglass CM stepwedge consisting of 10 cuvettes 1 cm in width containing the following percentage dilutions of Angiografin: 2, 4, 6, 8, 10, 20, 30, 40, 50, and 60. At the end of the stepwedge was an area of flat water-filled cuvettes which represented the background signal for calibration.

The investigation was carried out with standard roentgenologic equipment (roentgen apparatus: Pantoskop, Siemens; image intensifier: RBV 23/13 caesium iodide, Siemens; video-television chain: Video med 3, Siemens; videorecorder; Sirecord XS, Siemens). The videodensitometer (G2027, Siemens) has been described in detail by *Lissner* and *Marhoff* (1968).

Measurement I: The CM stepwedge was led through the bundle of radiation under the following conditions: 75 kV, 2 mA; filtration with 6 mm Al and 0.5 mm Cu. The density values of the stepwedge were depicted on an oscilloscope using the horizontal lines of the video image behind the logarithm integrator and were then drawn from the screen of the oscilloscope.

Measurement II: This was principally the same as measurement I, but in order to intensify the radiation scattering a water layer with a thickness of 13 cm was positioned in the path of the X-rays.

2.3 Results

The output voltages which corresponded to the various concentrations of the CM were determined by calibration curves. Apart from the highest CM concentration value, our measuring system shows a linear curve of the overall function (Fig. 3a). The influence of the scattering object is shown in Fig. 3b, where a little nonlinearity was observed over the whole measured range of CM concentrations even after conversion to logarithms.

2.4 Discussion

Our investigation demonstrates that the output signal of our X-ray–television chain, including the densitometer and the logarithmic converter, varies nearly linearly with the CM concentration and that therefore our conventional X-ray equipment has for practical purposes sufficient accuracy in densitometric measurements. The applicability of the Lambert-Beer law in roentgen-densitometry through the use of adequate filtering, and the necessity to convert the video voltage by video amplifiers with excellent logarithmic characteristics, has been widely discussed (*Bürsch* et al. 1969; *Hilal* 1966; *Heintzen* 1971; *Rutishauser* 1969). Less attention, however, has been paid to the influence of Compton scattering on densitometric measurements. Compton scattering not only impairs the contrast by increasing the background radiation, but also interferes with the densitometric measurement if the scattered X-rays transit the CM in the direction of the input screen of the image intensifier. Our second measurement, with a scattering object, shows the influence of radiation scattering through a small nonlinearity of the logarithmic extinction curve. The Compton scattering which arises unavoidably in the patient partly offsets the homogenizing effect of the filtering, so that strictly speaking the conditions of the Lambert-Beer law are not met. For the determination of the transit time of a CM bolus

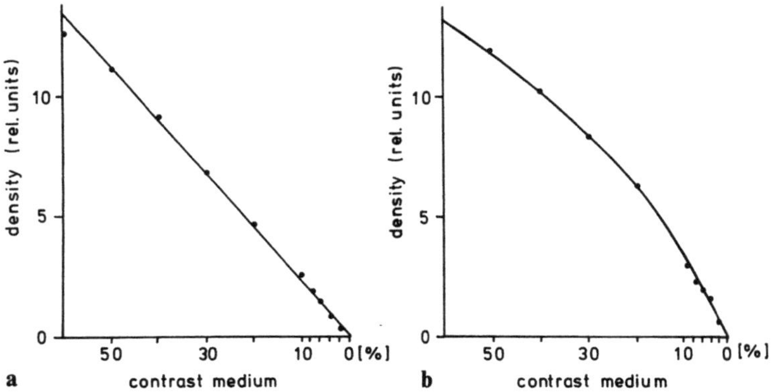

Fig. 3a, b. The logarithmically converted density signals in proportion to the concentration of CM. **a** For practical experimental conditions there is a linear transfer function of the X-ray–television chain and densitometer. **b** There is a slightly curvilinear course of the density curve due to X-ray scattering when a water column is exposed to radiation

between two measuring points, only the definition of the relative CM concentration is necessary. Therefore the error due to a small nonlinearity of the transfer function is negligibly small, as long as the two CM concentration curves are subject to the same nonlinear deviation and the concentration differences are not too great (*Brennecke* et al. 1983).

3 Developing an Analyzing Unit

3.1 Introduction

In our opinion there exists no satisfactory technical means which can be used for a quantitative analysis of CM density curves. The method used by *Rutishauser* (1969) – cutting the CM density curves out of paper and determining the lines of gravity by balancing the curve on the edge of a knife – cannot enter into routine clinical measuring procedure. In order to calculate the density curves with the central computer of a hospital, a very special interface of data transmission has to be developed. Utilization of smaller, decentralized computers of the PDP 11 type, together with associated equipment, requires a well-trained programming and computer operating staff. In the past few years digital processing of video-angiograms has been increasingly applied to blood flow measurement in radiology. This technique is still in the developmental stage (*Bürsch* et al. 1981); however, in our opinion the high cost of the systems for digital image processing is not satisfactory in relation to the diagnostic meaningfulness of a blood flow measurement. This problem of cost-benefit analysis is perhaps an important reason why videodensitometric measurements have not been implemented as part of routine angiographic examinations. It was our aim to develop a method of evaluation which fulfills the following practical conditions: (a) low prime costs; (b) low maintenance costs by avoiding the need for specialist operating and programming staff; (c) ease of comprehension and operation by auxiliary medical staff; (d) the ability to perform different quantitative analyses (line-of-gravity method, cross-correlation function).

3.2 Description of Our Analyzing System

A number of suitable, reasonably priced microcomputers, which in the past few years have found wide usage because of their universal application, were on offer. We used a personal computer, the Commodore CBM 3032, which has a monitor with high spatial resolution display and an ASCII keyboard.

The CBM 3032 system can be programmed easily with the versatile programming language Basic. In addition it is possible to write the program directly in the assembler language of the microprocessor. This method considerably increases the rate at which processing takes place, and we used it for quick transfer of data. To save learning a programming language, we developed the programming sequence as a form of dialogue.

For the input of analog voltage from the videodensitometer we developed an interface with two analog-to-digital (AD) converters. Digitalization and input of the

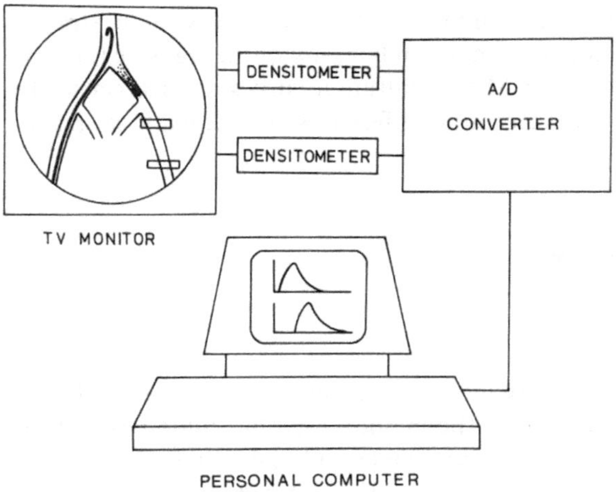

Fig. 4. Principle of videodensitometric analysis unit with a personal computer

densitometer curves through the two AD converters in the computer are regulated through a multiplex system. After the data transfer, the densitometer curves are displayed within a coordinate system on the monitor and are ready to be analyzed (Fig. 4). Parameters such as the diameter of the vessel or the distance from the measuring windows can also be fed into the computer if required.

Three different algorithms can be used to calculate Δt from the two densitometer curves. For the calculation of the line of gravity $\bar{t}$ of a homogeneous area under the curve $c = f(t)$ the following equation applies:

$$\bar{t} = \frac{\int_{t_0}^{t\infty} C \cdot (t) \cdot t \cdot dt}{\int_{t_0}^{t\infty} C \cdot (t) \cdot dt} \tag{4}$$

$\bar{t}$ is calculated from each curve; then $\bar{t}_2 - \bar{t}_1 = \Delta t$ follows.

Through digitalization of the two densitometer curves, equidistant points on the curves are given so that for the integration, an approximation method – the trapeze rule – offers itself. After the input of the diameter of the vessel and its length Δl, the transit time Δt (ms) and the blood flow velocity (cm/s) and volume (ml/min) are displayed on the monitor.

The position of the line of gravity is decisively influenced by the later part of the curve, which often does not decrease to the zero-line. The reason for this is considered to be the incomplete mixing of CM and blood due to the viscosity and gravity of the CM (*Heuck* et al. 1975). In the analysis, therefore, the zero-line of the curve must be defined by the investigator starting with the end of the curve. In this way the operator can set the zero-line on the monitor.

In order to be able to estimate the influence of the slope at the end of the curve upon the results from the line-of-gravity method, we modify the calculating method in such a way that only a preset percentage of the signal amplitude enters the calculation. The computer, starting with the highest value of the curve (100%), fixes the zero-line at a height of 10% of the maximum of the curve if the starting percentage

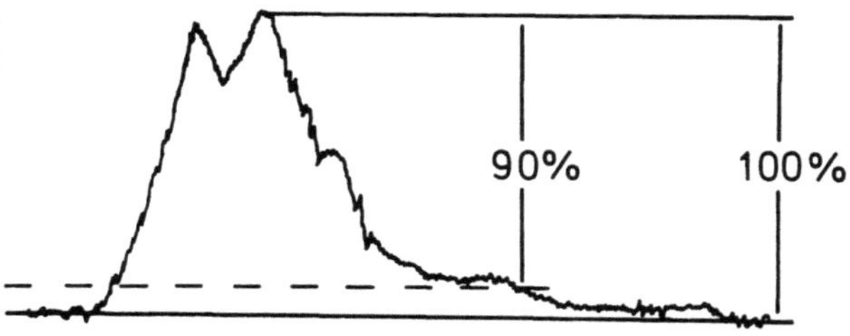

Fig. 5. Method to estimate the influence of the slope of the densitometer curve on the calculated flow volumes (see text)

value is for instance 90% (Fig. 5). Only the curve values above the new zero-line will be used to determine the line of gravity.

The cross-correlation function $F_{1,2}$ [Eq. (3)] is a measure of the statistical dependence of two stationary processes. The computer-calculated cross-correlation function for the two densitometer curves in Fig. 6a is shown in Fig. 6b. In order to determine the complete cross-correlation function for the given length of densitometer curves, over 200,000 multiplications and additions have to be performed, for which the microcomputer takes an unacceptably long time. For the determination of the transit time however, the calculation of the complete cross-correlation is unnecessary: only the maximum value, that is the moment of maximum overlap, is of interest.

The investigator can, by estimating the temporal distance between the maximal values of the curves, roughly assess the maximal position of the cross-correlation function. This position is fed to the computer, which consequently only needs to

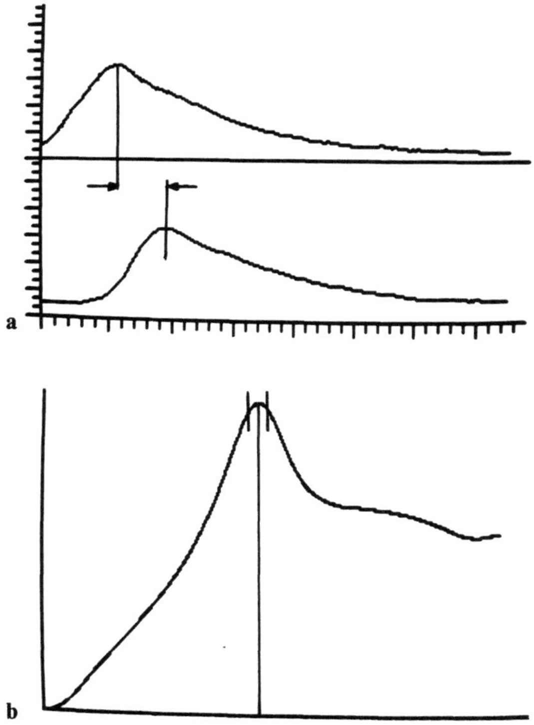

Fig. 6a, b. Photograph from the computer monitor. For the two densitometer curves (**a**) the cross-correlation function (**b**) is calculated (relative units). A section around the maximum of the cross-correlation function which is of interest for the calculation of Δt can roughly be estimated from the temporal distance of the densitometric curve maxima

calculate the cross-correlation within given parameters around the stated maximal value in order to determine the real maximal value. In this way the calculation time can be reduced to a few minutes. Control programs ensure that errors in the position of the maximal point are indicated to the investigator. After input of the vessel parameters, the flow velocity and volume are calculated as shown above.

4 Experimental Videodensitometric Blood Flow Measurement in Model Circulations

4.1 Introduction

Even though the accuracy of densitometric measurement has been verified in model circulations by several authors (*Bürsch* et al. 1971; *Decker* et al. 1973; *Femor* et al. 1979; *Rutishauser* 1969; *Rutishauser* et al. 1970), we consider further model circulation investigations necessary in order to examine the following problems:

1. The investigations by the authors quoted were mostly performed using cinedensitometry. Because of the greater temporal resolution of cinedensitometry, the results in connection with the special technical requirement for high voltage stabilization (*Heintzen* 1971) can only with reservations be compared with the results from a videodensitometric measuring apparatus. We therefore had to answer the question of whether a conventional roentgen apparatus is suitable for videodensitometric blood flow measurements of sufficient precision.
2. We consider model measurements to be valuable when situations encountered in clinical practice are simulated. Since we were interested in the blood flow into the lower extremity, we carried out experiments with a model vessel equivalent in its dimensions to the arteria iliaca externa. Flow volumes were created similar to those which exist in vivo. We wished to include the influence of unavoidable X-ray scattering in the human body on our measurements, as well as the influence of the inhomogeneous background of the object.
3. Systematic investigations of the influence of the quantity of CM injected upon the flow measurements are not to be found in the literature. Due to the greater viscosity of CM relative to blood and its higher specific gravity, deviations in measurement are conceivable.
4. It has to be determined which of the mathematicl analyses discussed gives the greatest accuracy in determining blood flow.
5. In our opinion the most important problem of densitometric blood flow analysis – the influence of the pulsation of flow on measurement – should be described.

We investigated problems 1–4 with a continuous flow model; for problem 5 a pulsating flow model was used.

4.2 Model Experiments with Continuous Flow

4.2.1 Method

Pig blood diluted with a calcium citrate solution was run from a reservoir through a 7-mm-diameter polyethylene tube into a lower receptacle. The volumetric blood flow (V_V) was varied with a tube clamp and measured with a stopwatch and measuring cylinder. The CM (Angiografin 65%) was injected with a power injector Contrac 3 (Contrave), at a sufficient distance upstream from the flow measuring section. In this way the velocity of the CM appearing in the measuring section could not be influenced by the injection velocity (10 ml/s) of the syringe. A container with 13 cm water served as a scattering body. The X-rays (75 kV, 2.5 mA) were filtered with 6 mm Al and 0.5 mm Cu. The automatic control of the video camera was set on a constant light value. In order to take measurements with an inhomogeneous background, we installed a 1.5-cm layer of plexiglass in the measuring section of one sampling window.

The following measurements were taken during continuous flow:

Series A

a) The blood flow was varied in the range 100–2000 ml/min, a degree of variation similar to that occurring in pelvic arteries
b) Injection of 1, 2, 3, and 5 ml CM (Angiografin 65%)
c) Analysis of CM density curves by the line-of-gravity method with 100%, 90%, and 80% signal parts, as well as by the cross-correlation method
d) Analysis by the line-of-gravity method, with a plexiglass layer positioned in one sampling window (CM boli 1 and 2 ml)

4.2.2 Results

For analysis of the model investigation, the influence of a great number of parameters upon the densitometrically determined flow V_D (random variable) have to be investigated in relation to the volumetric flow V_V. Since the volumetric blood flow is independent, the deviations of the random variables resulting from the parameters cannot be determined through a multivariate analysis. We therefore evaluated the connection between densitometric and volumetric flow values through correlation functions. The correlation coefficient (r), the standard deviation ($S_{y,x}$), the slope of the regression curve (b) if $V_V = x$, and the axial section (a) on the ordinate if $x = 0$ were compiled in tables, since the large number of correlation analyses could not all be depicted graphically. If one compares the stated functions, then one can estimate the influence of the varying parameters in the model on the accuracy of the results. From the increase of the zero point regression line, one can calculate the systematic estimation error (SE) under consideration by comparing, in pairs, the volumetric to the videometric results.

After analysis with the line-of-gravity method and 100% curve amplitude (Table 1a), we find, with a CM bolus of 2 ml, the maximal correlation coefficient, the lowest standard deviation, and the smallest SE of 0%–5%. With increasing CM volume the correlation coefficient diminishes and the standard deviation increases slightly. If one calculates the density curves by the line-of-gravity method with a signal amplitude of 90%, then nearly all correlation coefficients increase compared with those of the 100% amplitude analysis (Table 1b). The standard deviations decrease accordingly. After analysis with 80% signal amplitude, the correlation coefficients hardly change at all (Table 1c). In addition we calculated the mean values of flow volumes which resulted from the analysis with signal amplitudes of 100% and 90%, and correlated these mean values with the volumetric flow V_V (Table 1d). No increases in the correlation coefficients resulted.

Table 1. Correlation functions of densitometric vs volumetric flow: series A (continuous flow)

Analysis	CM (ml)	n	Corr. co.	$S_{y \cdot x}$	b	a	SE (%)
a)	1	26	0.982	116	0.932	41	-6.8*
Line of gravity	2	26	0.986	92	0.951	71	-4.9
100% sig. ampl.	3	26	0.982	106	0.956	-78	-4.4
	5	21	0.978	103	0.895	-76	-10.5
b)	1	26	0.995	55	0.963	7	-3.7
Line of gravity	2	26	0.992	71	1.0	-96	0
90% sig. ampl.	3	26	0.99	77	0.960	-71	-4
	5	21	0.933	204	0.970	-105	-3
c)	1	26	0.996	54	0.975	10	-2.5
Line of gravity	2	26	0.991	70	1.0	-55	0
80% sig. ampl.	3	26	0.991	70	0.950	-76	-5
	5	21	0.98	86	0.935	-85	-6.5
d)	1	26	0.994	70	0.947	39	-5.3
Line of gravity	2	26	0.993	69	0.977	-69	-2.3
100% + 90% sig. ampl.							
e)	2[a]	26	0.989	83	0.88	17	-12
Line of gravity							
100% sig. ampl.							
f)	1	26	0.993	65	0.922	113	-7.8
Cross-correlation	2	26	0.988	138	0.897	197	-10.3

CM, CM bolus of 1–5 ml Angiografin
* Inhomogeneous background

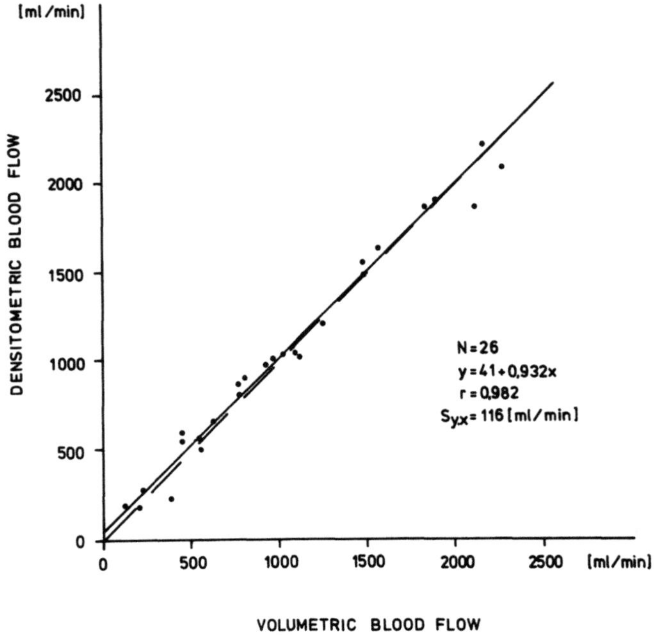

Fig. 7. Typical correlation diagram of volumetric vs densitometric flow (indicated in Table 1a with asterisks)

Table 1c shows the relations for the measurements taken with an inhomogeneous background. Here we also find a good correlation. Analysis with cross-correlation gives better results after injection of 1 ml CM than after injection of 2 ml CM boli. The systematic error (SE) is about 10% (Table 1f). One example of a typical correlation diagram has been given in Fig. 7.

4.2.3 Discussion

The results show that flow values which were determined through the use of conventional X-ray equipment with a videodensitometer and an analysis system we developed, correlate favorably with the volumetrically measured flow values. In the literature (*Bürsch* et al. 1971; *Decker* et al. 1973; *Femor* et al. 1979) we find similarly high correlation coefficients for a continuous circuit model. A systematic investigation of the effect of the amount of CM injected on the accuracy of measurements has not yet emerged. Some authors (*Decker* et al. 1973; *Piroth* et al. 1979) merely specify the injected CM quantity of 1.5–2 ml, or are content with the general statement that preferably small quantities of CM should be used. This view is confirmed by our findings. A large quantity of CM does not mix as well with the blood stream and, through sedimentation, causes a delayed descending slope of the CM density curve. In our model circuit, CM boli of 5 ml resulted in an underestimation of blood flow by about 10% in the analysis with 100% signal amplitude, and by about 3% with 90% signal amplitude.

However, it remains to be stated that with all chosen CM boli the correlation coefficients are significant and vary only minimally. Large errors of analysis should not be expected to result from too large or too small CM boli. For practical applications it is sufficient to ensure a short CM bolus with adequate contrast by making a test injection.

If one compares the mathematical analyses, one finds the most significant correlation coefficients and the smallest systematic errors using the line-of-gravity method with either 90% and 80% signal amplitude, thereby eliminating the sedimentation parts of the curve. The use of a mean value of flow volume calculated from 100% and 90% signal amplitudes does not improve the resultant correlation functions.

A good correlation is found with cross-correlation analysis, whose accuracy, however, is influenced by the shape of the curve maximum. With a CM bolus of 2 ml, the correlation with volumetric blood flow through the flat maximum of the curve is not as good as with a short bolus of 1 ml, which gives a sharper top of the curve. With an inhomogeneous background the intensity and the quality of X-rays are not identical in both sampling windows. Both curves are subject to an unavoidable nonlinear distortion, which can affect them to varying degrees. Our investigation with an inhomogeneous background, in the form of a plexiglass layer in the path of the X-rays at one sampling window, does not show significant deviation in the correlation of V_D with V_V as compared to measurements with a homogeneous background.

In conclusion, we can say that blood flow volumes with continuous flow can be measured using a conventional X-ray apparatus and a videodensitometer, with an error of about – 5% which depends on the size of CM bolus, the type of mathematical analysis, and the homogeneity of the background.

4.3 Influence of Pulsating Flow on Densitometric Determinations

4.3.1 Introduction

The videodensitometric measurement of continuous blood flow, as stated, gives a very exact result. The question remains as to whether this precision of measurement will be also achieved if – as is the case in the large arterial vessels – the blood flow is pulsating. In measuring a pulsating flow, the following velocities must be taken into account (*Vanselow* et al. 1975):

1. The instantaneous velocity: the speed at a given instant of a single particle within the vessel.
2. The mean flow velocity: the speed of which the blood or CM bolus moves through several pulsation cycles.
3. The front velocity: the speed with which the front of a CM bolus spreads in the direction of the flow.
4. The pulse-wave velocity: the speed with which the pulse moves through the vessel, also called the phase velocity.

The CM blood which has been accelerated by the pulse wave has a lower velocity than the pulse wave itself, which moves through the discontinuously flowing medium with the phase velocity *P*. Between the wave maxima the CM bolus has a very low velocity. If the CM bolus is very small compared with the wavelength, then it represents the instantaneous velocity of a blood particle (Fig. 8 a). In reality, the ideal small CM bolus, on mixing with the blood, is subject to increasing spreading so that the velocity of the bolus is influenced at the same moment by different cycle phases (Fig. 8 b). The CM moves over a greater distance of several cycle lengths with a mean flow velocity *G*. In a broad CM bolus, the front velocity *F* is the same as the instantaneous velocity over the point of measurement. As long as the length of the CM bolus represents one cycle length or a multiple of one cycle length, then the sum of the instantaneous velocities coincides with the mean flow velocity *G* of a cycle. From the temporal shifting (Δt) of the CM density curves and the distance between the measuring points (Δl), the blood flow velocity can be determined. With a hypothetical small measuring distance, m_1 to m_2 (Fig. 8 b), and a short CM bolus (compared with the cycle length), only the instantaneous velocity from a section of the cycle will be measured. From the measuring positions depicted it is not possible to determine the mean front velocity or the mean flow velocity. If however the distance between the two measuring points m_3 and m_4 in Fig. 8 b is a large one, then within the measuring section there lies the whole range of different instantaneous blood velocities of a cycle. With this measurement, the front velocity or the mean flow velocity can be determined.

However, the anatomic construction of arteries often only allows a choice of small measuring sections, because long nonbranching vessel sections cannot be found. *Vanselow* et al. have therefore recommended, for the determination of the mean front or mean flow velocities, a real-time sampling method, in which from discrete measurement values *I* are determined from instantaneous blood flow velocities during several cycles. Here one proceeds as follows: Several CM boli are injected successively from a cycle-controlled syringe. The moment of injection in each case is shifted with the time span *s* or a multiple of *s* (Fig. 9 a). From the discrete measure-

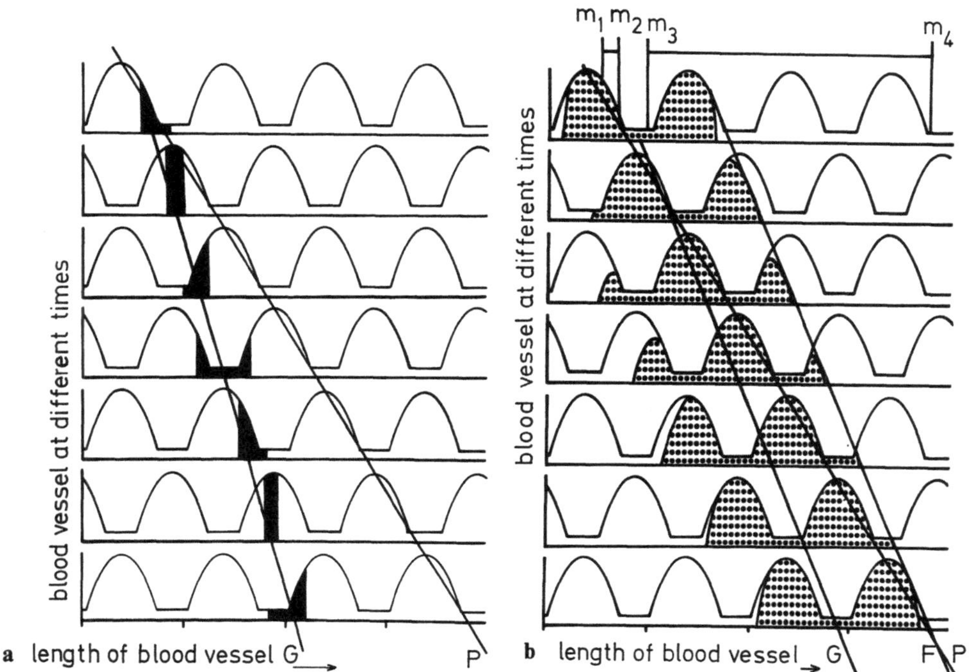

Fig. 8a, b. The pulse wave passes through the circulating blood and CM with the phase velocity *P* (modified after Vanselow et al.). **a** The mean flow velocity *G* of an ideal small CM bolus represents the instantaneous velocity of blood particles. **b** A broad CM bolus is influenced at the same time by different cycles with the mean flow velocity *G*. The front velocity (*F*) represents the instantaneous velocity of blood flow

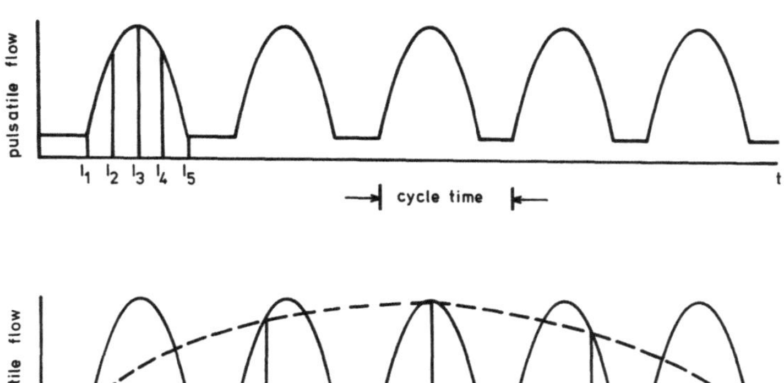

Fig. 9. Principle of the real-time sampling method. The whole spectrum of velocity distributions of a cycle can be found by the discrete measurement values I_1–I_5 (*upper panel*), which also can be taken from different cycles (*lower panel*). (Modified after Vanselow et al.)

ment values $I_1, I_2, I_3 \ldots$ one finds the whole spectrum of velocity distributions of a cycle (Fig. 9b). Strictly speaking, by densitometry one cannot determine the instantaneous velocity I at an exact moment, but only a mean velocity between two points within the time Δt Eq. (2). Therefore the interval s between two discrete measurements value I should be the same as Δt. In this case the discrete measurement values I correspond to transittimes, with which the mean flow velocities of the cycle can be determined. This ideal method of densitometric flow measurement cannot however be utilized, since Δt is not known before the measurement is taken. The front velocity is equivalent to an instantaneous velocity. But only the front velocity of a bolus can be used for the calculation of Δt by the real-time sampling method if this ideal condition is given. If however Δt is determined with the line-of-gravity method, then the mean flow velocity of the bolus enters the measurements. One can therefore assume that false measurements of mean flow velocity of a cycle, through the choice of too small or too large intervals s in relation to the length of the CM bolus, can be minimized. The aim of our investigation, through simulation of our chosen clinical measuring conditions, was to determine both the number of CM boli per cycle and the measuring intervals s, in order to achieve exact densitometric flow values with the real-time sampling method.

The model circulation for pulsating flow quoted in the literature (*Decker* et al. 1973; *Femor* et al. 1979) does not in our opinion simulate the circulation in the greater arteries. The quoted authors used exclusively the roller pump normally used for hemodialysis, which creates an almost sinusoidal phasic flow (Fig. 10). A phasic flow thus created does not correspond to the phasic flow found in the great main arteries. With an intravascular ultrasonic flowmeter, we registered the instantaneous blood flow velocity in the external iliac artery (arteria iliaca externa) of five patients and found the typical velocity distribution shown in Fig. 11, with an initial short increase of velocity followed by a sharp decrease. After this the blood flowed at a lower speed. In old patients the decrease may even reach negative values i.e., a backflow.

4.3.2 Method

In order to simulate a physiological velocity distribution, we used a piston pump (Alldos KM234) with which the output volume and the output stroke could be proportionally regulated through a drive. For our measurements we first created an amplitude of 70% (Fig. 12a), and then an amplitude of 100% with a backflow

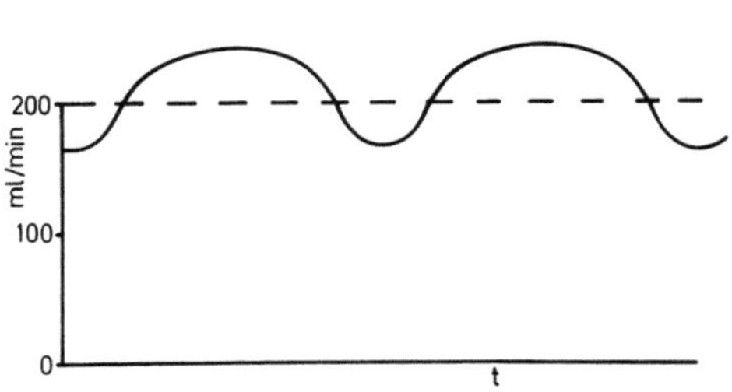

Fig. 10. Typical curves of instantaneous flow after the flow model of *Femor* et al. (1979). A small sinusoidal pulsation is superimposed on a high constant flow. Accordingly, the CM bolus is mainly transported through the constant flow

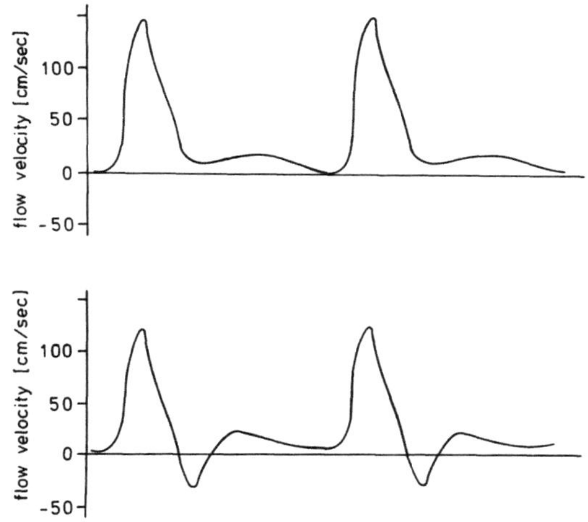

Fig. 11. Typical velocity distributions in the arteria iliaca externa. *Upper panel:* 30-year-old patient; *lower panel:* 75-year-old patient

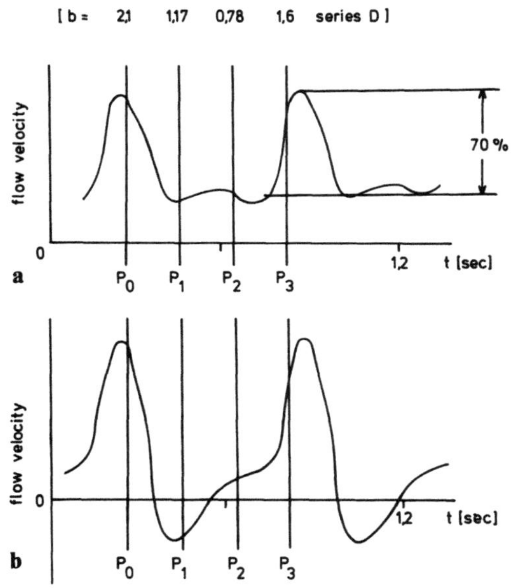

Fig. 12 a, b. Velocity distribution of blood flow model with pulsatile flow. **a** Amplitude is 70% of maximum of flow velocity. **b** Amplitude is 100% of maximum of flow velocity and there is a backflow. P_0–P_3, injection points of CM boli

(Fig. 12 b). Comparison between our simulated velocity distribution and the physiological velocity distribution showed a large degree of conformity. The cycle frequency was 100/min. The model is shown in Fig. 13. The setting of the X-ray equipment corresponds to that in the continuous flow model. In order to register the instantaneous velocity of the pulsating flow, we used a bidirectional ultrasonic device after *Borgnis* (*Borgnis* and *Frutiger* 1969). The steeply rising flanks of the curve of flow velocity which were registered by the ultrasonic device were used for triggering the CM injection. The trigger impulse for the power injector corresponds to a phase of the cycle at the points P_0, P_1, P_2, and P_3 (Fig. 12 a). Before each injection, the phase position of the trigger impulse was adjusted using its reference signal on a two-beam oscilloscope. In subsequent series we used this blood flow model to investigate the relationship between the flow volume obtained by densitometry and the volumetrically measured blood flow.

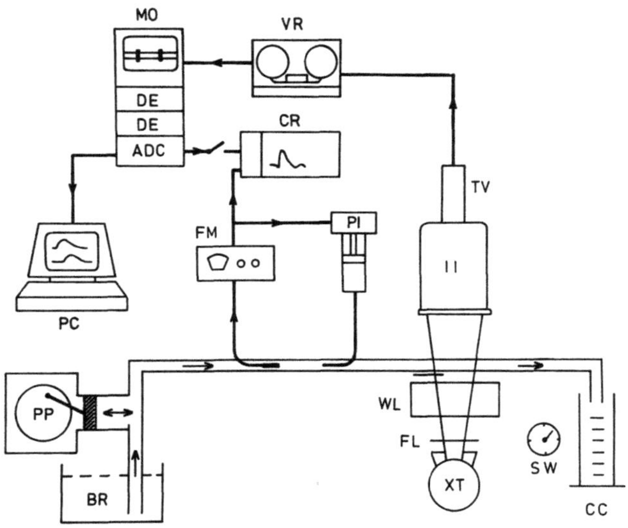

Fig. 13. Model of pulsating blood flow. *XT*, X-ray tube; *FL*, filter; *WL*, water layer; *II*, image intensifier; *TV*, television camera; *VR*, video-tape recorder; *MO*, monitor; *DE*, densitometer; *ADC*, analog-digital converter; *PC*, personal computer; *CR*, chart recorder; *FM*, flowmeter; *PI*, power injector; *PP*, piston-metering pump; *BR*, blood reservoir; *CC*, cylinder; *SW*, stopwatch

Series B

a) Injection of 1–2 ml Angiografin 65%; variation of flow volumes 150–2200 ml/min
b) Flow amplitude of 70%
c) Four phase-triggered injection times, P_0–P_3
d) Analysis by the method of line of gravity with 100%, 90%, and 80% signal parts, as well as by cross-correlation

Series C

Measuring conditions as in Series B, but with 100% flow amplitude and backflow

4.3.3 Results

As in the analysis of the results from the continuous flow model, we tabulated the results of the correlation analyses of densitometric flow V_D against volumetric flow V_V. Densitometric flow volumes taken at the injection times P_0–P_3 of a phase cycle will be called V_{D0}–V_{D3}.

4.3.3.1 Dependence of Densitometric Flow Volumes on the Amplitude of Blood Flow

The correlation functions of the flow volumes V_{D0}–V_{D3} determined at the points P_0 to P_3 of a cycle have been recorded for series B and C in Tables 2 and 3. The flow values were calculated by the line-of-gravity method with a signal amplitude of 100%. The mean values of the correlation coefficients for V_{D0}–V_{D3} are distinctly

Table 2. Correlation functions of densitometric vs volumetric flow: series B (pulsating flow with 70% amplitude of flow; calculated after the line-of-gravity method; $n = 20$)

PI	Corr. co.	$S_{y \cdot x}$	b	a	SE (%)
P_0	0.915	288	1.29	−109	29
P_1	0.97	131	1.0	53	0
P_2	0.861	271	0.91	59	−9
P_3	0.923	241	1.15	−66	15
$\bar{x}$	0.917	232	1.08		8.8
SD	±0.044	±70	±0.16		±16

PI, point of injection of CM bolus at cycle times $P_0 - P_3$

Table 3. Correlation funtions of densitometric vs volumetric flow: series C (pulsating flow with 100% amplitude of flow and backflow; calculated after the line-of-gravity method; $n = 31$)

PI	Corr. co.	$S_{y \cdot x}$	b	a	SE (%)
P_0	0.875	422	1.4	−25	40
P_1	0.833	568	1.5	−216	50
P_2	0.767	329	0.68	340	−32
P_3	0.899	409	1.55	−176	55
$\bar{x}$	0.836	432	1.28		28
SD	±0.063	±98	±0.4		±40

higher in series B than in series C, the latter distinguishing itself from series B by a higher pulse amplitude and a backflow. The standard errors $S_{y.x}$ are smaller in series B than in series C.

4.3.3.2 Dependence of Densitometric Flow Volumes on the Cycle Phase

In the examples of typical density curves (Fig. 14), one can discern the length of the CM boli in relation to the pulse period of the flow velocity. The relationship of the length of bolus to the flow volume is shown graphically in Fig. 15. The length of bolus corresponds to the number of cycles through which the bolus extends. In the diagram the measurements for series B and series C have been combined, since the lengths of the CM boli were not unduly influenced by the flow amplitude. Starting with a bolus length calculated for a pulse rate of 100/min, we determined the length of the bolus for a pulse rate of 50/min. In the area between the two diagram curves, one can estimate the length of boli at a given flow volume for pulse rates between 100 and 50/min. Only values which were calculated, using the line-of-gravity method with 100% signal amplitude were considered.

In order to investigate the dependence of densitometric flow volumes upon the length of the CM boli, we calculated in series D the correlation function of $V_{D0} - V_{D3}$ for flow volumes of over 800 ml/min, at which the CM boli only covered a length of 1–3 cycles. The flow values for series D were taken from series B and C. The func-

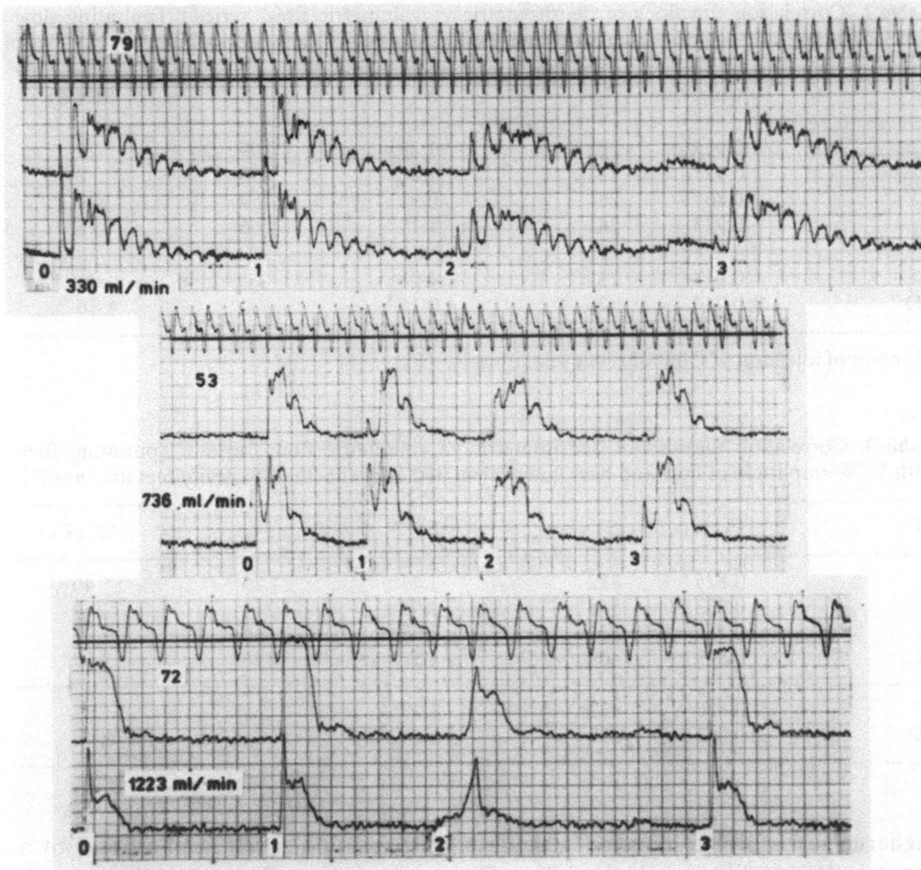

Fig. 14. Examples of typical CM density curves. Note the length of the CM boli in relation to the flow volume and the number of pulse periods (frequency 100/min, with backflow)

tions of series D are shown in Table 4a. The correlation coefficients were distinctly lower than in series B and C, because the range of variation of volumetric flow V_V was reduced. In series D, which is distinguished by short boli and high phasic velocity, we find a marked phasic dependence of the regression line gradient b at the injection points P_0–P_3. In order to underline the phasic over- and underestimation of the densitometric flow, we included the rise b of V_{D0}–V_{D3} with the pulse cycle in Fig. 12. Rise b of the regression line at the systolic time P_0 reaches a value of 2.1; that is, V_{D0} is determined as 110% higher than the mean volumetric flow. In comparison, rise b at the late diastolic time P_2, is 0.78, i.e. V_{D2} is underestimated by 22%.

Obviously, one cannot measure the real flow with a densitometric flow volume which has been determined for only one point in the cycle. We therefore calculated for series D, according to the real-tine sampling method, the mean values for the flow at the injection points P_0–P_3 with the following combinations: $V_{D0}+V_{D1}$; $V_{D0}+V_{D2}$; $V_{D0}+V_{D3}$; $V_{D1}+V_{D2}$; $V_{D1}+V_{D3}$; $V_{D2}+V_{D3}$; $V_{D0}+V_{D1}+V_{D2}$; $V_{D0}+V_{D2}+V_{D3}$; $V_{D0}+V_{D1}+V_{D3}$; $V_{D1}+V_{D2}+V_{D3}$; $V_{D0}+V_{D1}+V_{D2}+V_{D3}$.

Fig. 15. The relation of the length of the CM bolus to flow volume. The length of the bolus corresponds to the number of cycles through which the bolus extends

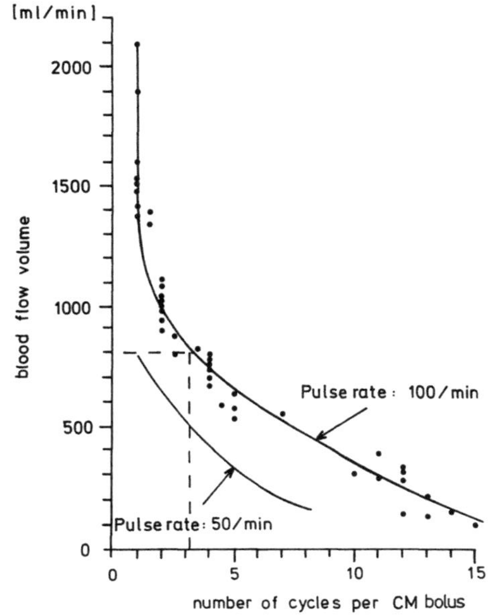

Table 4. Correlation functions of densitometric vs volumetric flow: series D (pulsating flow values over 800 ml/min; calculated after the line-of-gravity method; $n=22$)

	PI	Corr. co.	$S_{y \cdot x}$	b	a	SE (%)
a)	P_0	0.751	484	2.1	−1193	110
	P_1	0.609	598	1.17	254	17
	P_2	0.615	323	0.78	175	−22
	P_3	0.703	523	1.6	−432	60
	$\bar{x}$	0.669	481	1.41		41
	SD	±0.069	±115	±0.56		±56
b)	P_0+P_1	0.891	410	1.48	−120	48
	P_0+P_2	0.902	270	1.0	157	0
	P_0+P_3	0.928	322	1.48	−100	48
	P_1+P_2	0.859	363	1.13	62	13
	P_1+P_3	0.899	411	1.56	−196	56
	P_2+P_3	0.917	263	1.11	81	11
	$\bar{x}$	0.899	399	1.29		29
	SD	±0.023	±65	±0.024		24
c)	$P_0+P_1+P_2$	0.903	313	1.21	33	21
	$P_0+P_2+P_3$	0.938	243	1.21	46	21
	$P_0+P_1+P_3$	0.919	349	1.5	−139	50
	$P_1+P_2+P_3$	0.91	313	1.26	−17	26
	$\bar{x}$	0.917	304	1.29		29
	SD	±0.015	±44	±0.14		±14
d)	$P_0+P_1+P_2+P_3$	0.926	286	1.3	−19	30

The relationship of these mean flow values to the volumetric flow V_V has been collated in Table 4b–d. If one considers the mean flow volumes from two CM bolus injections ($V_{D0}+V_{D1}$ ...) then one finds in all mean value combinations higher correlation coefficients than those values taken from one flow measurement of the cycle. In the same way, the standard error of estimation $S_{y.x}$ decreases. It is also striking that in Table 4b, for all value combinations which incorporate V_{D2}, the rise b of the regression line is very close to 1. From this combination one finds the least over- or underestimation compared with the real volumetric flow. If one calculates the mean values from the densitometric flow volumes measured at three or four points of the cycle then the correlation coefficients increase in all combinations, while $S_{y.x}$ decreases. The rise b of the regression line does not vary to the same degree. There is however no measurement of b which is less than 1.2; this means that from the mean values of the flow volumes from three to four measuring points, an overestimation of at least 20% arises.

4.3.3.3 Relationship of Flow Volume Values to the Method of Analysis

We calculated the flow volumes V_{D0}–V_{D3} by the line-of-gravity method with 90% and 80% signal amplitude, and correlated these with V_V. The functions of correlation have been collated in Tables 5 and 6. In series B the correlation coefficients with a 90% or 80% utilization of signal amplitude (Table 5) are distinctly greater

Table 5. Correlation functions of densitometric vs volumetric flow: series B (pulsating flow with 70% amplitude of flow; $n=20$)

Analysis	PI	Corr. co.	$S_{y \cdot x}$	b	a	SE (%)
a)	P_0	0.95	201	1.22	−130	22
Line of gravity	P_1	0.95	173	1.0	16	0
90% sig. ampl.	P_2	0.948	148	0.88	35	−12
	P_3	0.94	212	1.17	−87	17
	$\bar{x}$	0.947	183	1.07		7
	SD	±0.04	±28	±0.16		±15
b)	P_0	0.965	216	1.23	−139	23
Line of gravity	P_1	0.935	167	1.14	−38	14
80% sig. ampl.	P_2	0.964	129	0.93	6	−7
	P_3	0.937	239	1.3	−134	30
	$\bar{x}$	0.95	187	1.15		15
	SD	±0.016	±49	±0.16		±16
c)	P_0	0.955	169	1.07	116	7
Cross-correlation	P_1	0.917	321	1.12	16	12
	P_2	0.873	223	0.89	43	−11
	P_3	0.943	188	0.93	−56	−7
	$\bar{x}$	0.922	188	1.00		0
	SD	±0.036	±24	±0.11		±11

Table 6. Correlation functions of densitometric vs volumetric flow: series C (pulsating flow with 100% amplitude of flow and backflow; $n=31$)

Analysis	PI	Corr. co.	$S_{y \cdot x}$	b	a	SE (%)
a)	P_0	0.901	334	1.2	−32	20
Line-of-gravity	P_1	0.855	450	1.3	−143	30
90% sig. ampl.	P_2	0.697	406	0.72	316	−28
	P_3	0.91	304	1.23	−216	23
	$\bar{x}$	0.84	573	1.11		11
	SD	±0.098	±66	±0.27		±27
b)	P_0	0.785	587	1.37	−85	37
Line-of-gravity	P_1	0.823	584	1.56	−224	56
80% sig. ampl.	P_2	0.533	672	0.77	371	−23
	P_3	0.829	396	1.08	105	8
	$\bar{x}$	0.724	559	1.19		19
	SD	±0.142	±116	±0.34		±34
c)	P_0	0.743	724	1.4	144	40
Cross-correlation	P_1	0.826	653	1.42	144	42
	P_2	0.643	542	0.71	93	−29
	P_3	0.893	623	1.02	−67	2
	$\bar{x}$	0.776	636	1.14		13
	SD	0.107	±80	±0.34		±34

than with a 100% utilization (Table 2), whereas in series C they remain constant with a 90% utilization and even decrease with an 80% utilization (Tables 3 and 6). The rises b of the regression lines of V_{D0}–V_{D3} relate to each other in the same way at a 90% or 80% utilization of signal amplitude as at a 100% utilization.

The correlation functions for V_{D0}–V_{D3} in series B (Table 5c) remain similar after cross-correlation, analogous to those of the line-of-gravity method with 100% signal amplitude. Only in series C (Table 6c) are the correlation coefficients at cross-correlation distinctly smaller, because with the high-velocity amplitude and backflow, the CM bolus changes in shape between the selected measuring points. The requirement for a cross-correlation measurement – the identical shape of the two density curves – therefore often does not exist. For this reason we dispensed with the calculation of mean flow volumes for V_{D0}–V_{D3}.

4.3.4 Discussion

Although several authors have already performed videodensitometric flow measurements on circulation models with periodically changing flow velocities as well as in animal experiments, the effect of a phase-dependent CM injection on the measurements has not yet been investigated systematically with a circulation model.

To date, *Pannek* et al. (1978) have been the only authors to use a real-time sampling method for videodensitometric flow measurements. They performed their investigations on aortocoronary bypass vessels whose real flow they did not know.

With a pulse-triggered bolus injection in the first, second, and third parts of a pulse cycle, they determined the mean front flow of a measuring interval and calculated the mean flow from the three flow measurements. The mean front velocity of a pulse phase can however only be determined exactly with this method if the total of the measured times of passage in all measuring sections comprises the period of a cycle. To fulfill this condition, the exact positioning of the trigger moments, the number of CM boli, and the cycle-dependent passage times Δt under investigation must be known before the measurement is taken. Our measurements of blood flow volumes in the area of the pelvic arteries show such high flow velocities and correspondingly short passage times of the bolus that with the method used by Pannek, four to eight phase-triggered bolus injections would have been necessary for the determination of blood flow.

According to *Pannek* et al. it is not possible to perform the calculation of mean velocity of a CM bolus with the real-time sampling method, since it cannot be equated with instantaneous flow. The objection is justified; however, it also applies, as stated above, to the front velocity. Obviously, an ideal evaluation method does not exist for measuring the pulsating blood flow with a CM bolus using the real-time sampling method. We chose the determination of mean velocity, i.e., mean transit time, since with this method the distribution of instantaneous velocities of the CM bolus enters the measurement results. One should therefore assume that with a smaller number of CM boli, the mean blood flow can be determined with real-time sampling.

Our measurement results show that with CM boli which extend across one to three pulse periods, the flow volumes determined with the line-of-gravity method or cross-correlation lead to a cycle-phase-dependent over- and underestimation of the real mean flow. This phenomenon is especially marked in the case of large flow amplitudes with a backflow.

Using the real-time sampling method, if we combine those flow volumes achieved through four CM injections over equidistant times in the cycle, then we find the best correlation results. However, this may produce a considerable overestimation of the densitometrically measured flow volumes, since the high systolic flow velocities are severally included. A similar situation arises with the determination of flow volumes using three CM boli. If one calculates the mean values of flow volumes from only two sampling points, then one finds in the mean value combinations which contain the diastolic flow V_{D2} the smallest over- or underestimations. The statement applies to flow velocities with high and low flow amplitudes, as well as to short and long (relative to the pulse period) CM boli.

It follows that for practical purposes, injection of one CM bolus at a systole and one at a diastole is adequate for a sufficiently exact densitometric flow measurement. The timing of a bolus at a systole or diastole is achieved when the phase-triggered injection points are staggered by half a cycle. The shifting of CM boli over a cycle phase on the route between injection point and measuring point obviously does not weigh so heavily, since the mean velocity also contains the distribution of the momentary velocities.

According to a diagram we produced, one can say as an approximation that the given interdependence of the mean velocities also applies at pulse frequencies smaller than 100/min.

It was demonstrated on a continuous flow model that the sedimentation of part of the contrast medium on the vessel floor leads to an undermeasurement of mean velocities. With a pulsating flow, high velocity can counteract the sedimentation. This effect can be demonstrated in our model investigation. In series B the flow amplitudes comprise only 70% of the maximum velocity. Therefore 30% of the flow remains continuous. If from the CM density curves of series B only the top 90% or 80% of signal amplitude is calculated with the line-of-gravity method, then the correlation coefficients of $V_{D0}-V_{D3}$ rise compared with the 100% amplitude calculation, in the mean from 0.917 to 0.951.

However, in series C, which has a velocity amplitude of 100% and a backflow, the mean correlation coefficients at 90% signal amplitude are just as great as with an analysis at 100% signal amplitude, and even decrease at an 80% signal amplitude.

The influence of the flow amplitudes of a pulsating flow on the accuracy of densitometric through-flow determination is also evident with cross-correlation calculations. Whereas in series B the mean correlation coefficient of $V_{D0}-V_{D3}$ (0.922) showed as good a correlation with volumetric flow as the calculation by the line-of- gravity method, in series C the mean correlation coefficient was only 0.776. Cross- correlation analysis requires that the CM density curves have almost identical shapes at both points of measurement. Through the high flow amplitudes, there arises in the course of the measuring section a considerable deformation of the second density curve, due to phase shifting between pulse and mean velocity, and therefore cross-correlation is not a suitable method of analysis for strong pulsating flows.

We conclude from the results of our investigations that there is no ideal method of calculation for densitometric blood flow measurement. The method of calculation should therefore be chosen according to the velocity profile of the blood flow. The course of the flow profile can as a rule be detected from the pulsation density changes of the measurement signals.

At high flow amplitudes we recommend the line-of-gravity method with 100% signal amplitude of the density curves to determine the densitometric through-flow. On the other hand, at relatively small amplitudes with a direct flow, either the line-of-gravity method with our modification of 90% amplitude measurement or cross-correlation should be chosen.

5 Videodensitometric Flow Measurements in the External Iliac Artery (Arteria Iliaca Externa)

5.1 Introduction

X-ray densitometric blood flow measurements have already been used by researchers in patients. *Rutishauser* (1969) measured the flow in the vena cava inferior, the arteria carotis, the aorta, and the coronary vessels. *Heuck* (*Heuck* 1973, 1983; *Heuck* et al. 1975) measured the blood flow in the arteria cerebri media and in the arteria renalis. Cinedensitometric flow measurements in the arteria iliaca externa have been made by *Itzchak* et al. (1975 a, b). The following clinical investigations were intended to evaluate the practical possibilities for using videodensitometric flow measurements on human pelvic vessels. We investigated the influence of pulsatile flow in the arteria iliaca externa on the densitometric blood flow measurements. Additionally we analyzed the CM density curves found in vivo, using diverse mathematical procedures. On a group of patients with arteriosclerosis obliterans, we measured densitometrically not only the blood flow at rest, but also the blood flow after ischemic work of the affected limb.

5.2 Blood Flow Measurement by Use of ECG-Triggered Injection of Contrast Medium

5.2.1 Method and Materials

According to our insight gained from the pulsating flow model, two CM boli injected at half-cycle intervals should be sufficient to determine the mean blood flow in the arteria iliaca with the real-time sampling method. In order to determine the variation in blood flow measurements due to a systolic or a diastolic CM injection, we measured in 13 patients, during the course of a pelvic, leg or renal arteriography, the flow volumes in the arteria iliaca externa by means of ECG-triggered CM injections. The tip of the catheter was introduced via a transfemoral or transaxillary entry, after Seldinger, just above the bifurcation into the aorta abdominalis. The CM quantities necessary for measurements were estimated through a trial injection. The complete passage of a CM bolus with good contrast should not exceed three cycles. As a rule we injected 3–5 ml Angiografin 65% at a velocity of 10 ml/s. The ECG signals and the trigger impulses of the high pressure syringe were displayed on a two-beam oscilloscope. With respect to the R-peak, the phase of the trigger impulse was shifted so that the injection followed at the time (T_1) of the systole (R-peak) or diastole (T_0; half cycle) respectively. The CM density curves were calculated by the line-of-gravity method and by cross-correlation.

In the group investigated (ten males, three females; mean age 60 years), nine patients had occlusive vascular disease of lower extremities. In one of these nine, the pelvic arteries were replaced by a Y-prosthesis, and in another the left arteria iliaca externa was replaced by a vessel prosthesis. Four patients who were examined later on by renal angiography showed no disturbed circulation of the lower extremities. Altogether, the blood flow in 14 arteria iliaca externa and three vessel grafts was measured. The vessel diameter was taken from an angiogram. By use of correction factors, we eliminated the magnifying effect due to the central projection of the X-rays.

5.2.2 Results

In Table 7 are shown the flow volumes as well as the mean transit times Δt in the arteria iliaca externa or vessel prostheses at systolic (T_1) and diastolic (T_2) injection points of the CM bolus. The values were calculated with the line-of-gravity method and 100% signal amplitude as well as with cross-correlation. The blood flow volumes (V_{T1}) taken at the injection point T_1 were compared with those (V_{T2}) taken at the injection point T_2 through correlation analysis (Fig. 16a, b). Disregarding for the correlation function those patients with a mean flow volume of over 800 ml/min,

Table 7. Individual values for blood flow and mean transit time (Δt) of the arteria iliaca externa

No.	Sex	Age	Side	Cal.	V_{T_1} (ml/min)	Δt (ms)	V_{T_2} (ml/min)	Δt (ms)	$\bar{V}$ (ml/min)	Condition
1.	M	75	L.	100%	325	600	218	898	271	Normal
				C. C.	235	830	232	840	233	
2.	M	50	L.	100%	555	274	499	306	527	ASO
				C. C.	637	240	546	280	591	
3.	M	48	R.	100%	390	542	541	390	465	Normal
				C. C.	406	520	431	490	418	
			L.	100%	401	616	443	557	422	
				C. C.	458	540	499	550	478	
4.	F	68	L.	100%	348	394	327	419	337	ASO
				C. C.	280	480	298	460	289	
5.	M	49	L.	100%	734	443	898	362	816	ASO
				C. C.	1302	250	1163	280	1235	
			R.	100%	489	211	586	173	542	Graft
				C. C.	646	160	760	140	703	
6.	M	66	L.	100%	653	499	797	409	725	Normal
				C. C.	742	440	772	420	757	
7.	M	50	L.	100%	716	659	1246	379	981	y-graft
				C. C.	760	690	690	760	725	
			R.	100%	860	503	816	530	836	
				C. C.	1237	350	883	490	1060	
8.	M	79	L.	100%	303	459	233	597	268	ASO
				C. C.	348	400	324	372	336	
9.	M	44	L.	100%	736	279	1278	161	1007	Normal
				C. C.	458	450	1623	113	1040	
10.	M	54	R.	100%	357	300	460	233	408	ASO
				C. C.	775	232	598	180	658	
11.	F	68	L.	100%	211	508	278	422	245	ASO
				C. C.	215	498	182	646	198	
12.	M	79	R.	100%	85	346	76	331	80	ASO
				C. C.	63	464	42	668	53	
13.	M	57	R.	100%	314	408	268	582	291	ASO
				C. C.	442	289	391	327	417	
			L.	100%	469	191	434	198	348	
				C. C.	538	190	440	197	489	

V_{T_1}/V_{T_2} flow volume measured with a systolic/diastolic injection of CM; Cal., method of calculation; C. C., cross-correlation; 100%, line-of-gravity method with 100% of signal amplitude; ASO, arteriosclerosis obliterans; Graft, vessel graft of the arteria iliaca externa; $\bar{V}$, mean of V_{T_1} and V_{T_2}.

the regression lines come close to the line of identity. The mean deviation between V_{T1} and V_{T2} in all 17 vessels examined was +40% by the line-of-gravity method and −20% by cross-correlation. If one considers only those vessels which by both calculation methods showed a mean flow of less than 800 ml/min, then the mean deviation between V_{T1} and V_{T2} narrowed after the line-of-gravity method to +6%, and after cross-correlation to −10%.

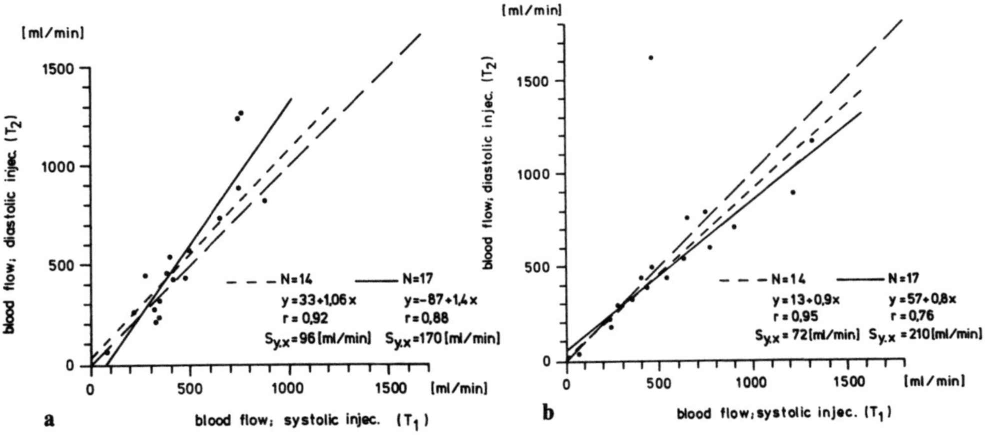

Fig. 16a, b. Correlation of densitometrically determined flow volumes in the arteria iliaca externa of human subjects measured with systolic and diastolic CM injections. **a** Analysis, by line-of-gravity method. **b** Analysis by cross-correlation. In the group $n=14$, only mean flow values of less than 800 ml/min are considered

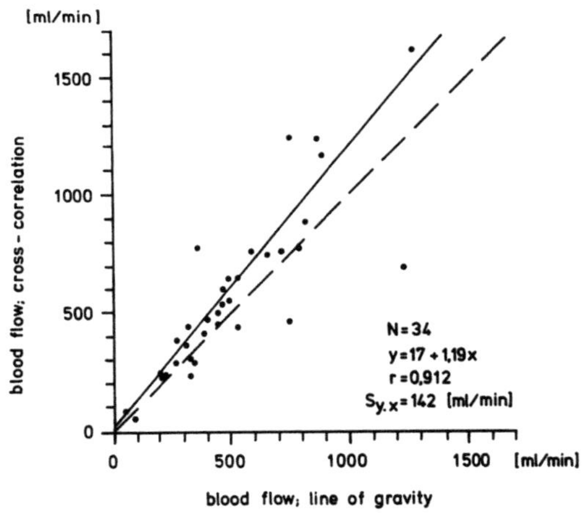

Fig. 17. The densitometrically determined flow volumes of the arteria iliaca externa (V_{T1} and V_{T2}) correlated after calculation with the line-of-gravity method and after cross-correlation analysis

The values for V_{T1} and V_{T2} after calculation with the line-of-gravity method and a 90% signal amplitude have been correlated and the correlation function reveals:

$$n=14; \quad y=9.5+1.09\,x; \quad r=0.915; \quad S_{y.x}=104 \text{ ml/min}$$

In a further correlation analysis, we examined the conformity of the flow values after calculating with the line-of-gravity method (100% signal amplitude) and after cross-correlation (Fig. 17).

5.2.3 Discussion

The flow values we recorded in the arteria iliaca externa were within a range equal to those found by other authors using cinedensitometric or other indicator-dilution methods (*Ganz* et al. 1964; *Itzchak* et al. 1975a, b; *Torfeldt* and *Wahren* 1971). However, it was not the aim of the present series of investigations to determine norms for normal or pathological flow values in the arteria iliaca externa by video-densitometry, but to analyze the degree of variation in flow volumes with consideration of the pulsating flow together with the various methods of mathematical evaluation. Unlike the measurements in flow models, the real flow values in the arteria iliaca externa are not known to us. In addition, exact timing of the flow velocities in the measuring section to a systole or a diastole is not possible with an ECG-triggered CM injection, since the mean flow time of the blood in the vessels prior to the arteria iliaca externa is not known. Therefore the influence of pulsating flow on the measurements can be judged through a comparison of flow measurements where the CM boli have been injected by triggering at different times of a cycle.

If one ignores high blood flow volumes, one finds that the blood flow of the arteria iliaca externa shows no remarkable systematic deviations dependent on the time of injection. As the correlation analyses show, the flow volumes determined at the point of time T_1 are either greater or slightly smaller than the flow measurements taken at the injection time T_2. A systematic deviation originates neither with calculation through the line-of-gravity method nor after cross-correlation. Therefore significant errors of measurement would not be expected with one simple CM injection if pulsatile blood flow is relatively low. ECG-triggered injections at systolic or diastolic points therefore give a higher measuring accuracy at low flow volumes, according to double measurements. If however one examines high flow volumes, as in the relatively young patient (No. 9 in Table 7), then according to the results from the flow volume models, the flow values taken at systolic or diastolic injection points can deviate considerably from each other. In these cases the phase-dependent injection cannot be considered as a simple double measurement, but as a quasi-real-time sampling technique in order to find the velocity distribution of a pulsatile flow.

In patients with vessel grafts we also find high flow measurements. These probably arise because the distal vessel connections, in addition to the femoral arteries, are connected through collateral arteries to other supply areas of the arteria iliaca interna.

In the realm of low flow measurements, no influence of pulsating flow on V_{T1} or V_{T2} is detectable. Here, the flow volumes which have been measured at two points of a cycle-phase-triggered CM injection correspond to a simple double measurement. On these twice-measured flow volumes, therefore, the reproducibility of flow measurements from in vivo CM density curves can be tested. We find the best reproduction, that is the highest correlation coefficient and the smallest standard error of estimation for V_{T1} vs V_{T2}, with cross-correlation analysis. Analysis by the line-of-gravity method with 100% or 90% signal amplitude gives correlation coefficients which are only slightly unfavorable.

In comparing the flow volumes determined by cross-correlation with those determined by the line-of-gravity method, we find a good correlation coefficient of 0.912. The values calculated with cross-correlation, however, are greater by about 19%.

Obviously there is a dependent relationship between the measured values of flow and the method of calculation chosen. For the practical clinical use of video-densitometric flow measurements, the present analyses have the following consequences: Since the flow volume and the range of amplitude of the pulsating flow are not known before a flow measurement has been made, one should generally inject two ECG-triggered CM boli at half-cycle intervals. Given a high flow volume and the gross difference between the two measured values because of the pulsating flow, then the mean value of the two measurements lies closer to the real flow value, because they are determined in accordance with the quasi-real-time sampling method. For low flow volumes, the mean value of both measurements represents the real flow as if in a double measurement.

In clinical investigations, the mathematical method of analysis used in the measurement of normal or pathological flow values should be stated, since, for example, a cross-correlation analysis may calculate flow volumes higher than the line-of-gravity method. Since videodensitometric measurements of absolute flow values depend on the method of analysis, we see a useful application of this method in the measurement of blood flow changes. A practical example would for instance be the measurement of flow increases in an extremity under stress. Cross-correlation can only be considered if the registered CM curves follow a nearly identical line over both measuring points. If this condition is not met, then the CM density curves should be calculated with the line-of-gravity method. For this we recommend that the flow volumes be measured with 100% and 90% signal amplitude. If these values differ considerably, then a disproportional influence of the curve ends exists in the results; in other words, the calculation of the flow volume is influenced by the CM sedimented in the vessel or spilled in the surrounding tissues. In this case the position of the measuring window or the volume of CM injected should be varied.

5.3 Flow Measurements in the Arteria Iliaca Externa in Patients with Arteriosclerosis Obliterans

5.3.1 Introduction

According to *Itzchak,* patients with arteriosclerosis obliterans (ASO) of lower extremities show a statistically lower mean densitometrically determined blood flow in the arteria iliaca externa than patients without vascular disease. There is considerable overlap in the binomial distributions, such that a distinction between pathological and normal flow is often not possible. This discovery coincides with the clinical observation that the majority of patients with ASO experience no discomfort at rest. Only under stress does the hypoxic pain force a discontinuance of muscle activity. We therefore regard it as reasonable to quantify the reduced active hyperemia with the help of videodensitometry, in the course of an angiography, without additional intervention. In a methodical study of a group of patients with ASO, we examined the practical application of videodensitometric flow measurements during exercise of the affected extremity.

5.3.2 Method and Materials

The investigations were conducted at a time when the instruments for ECG-triggered injections and computer analysis were not yet available. We therefore calculated the CM density curves graphically after the line-of-gravity method with 100% signal amplitude. The resulting restricted interpretations will be examined in the discussion.

In a total of 19 patients with ASO of Fontaine grade II–III, we measured the flow in the arteria iliaca externa following a maximum of exercise of the lower extremity. In 16 patients we were also able to measure the flow in the arteria iliaca externa on the unstressed side. The CM bolus (3–5 ml Angiografin 65%) was injected via a pig-tail catheter above the bifurcation in the aorta abdominalis.

In order to create active hyperemia we used the calf ergometer after Hildt, where the patient treads rhythmically with a frequency of 1/s against a pedal which raises a weight of 5 kp through a predetermined distance of 0.3 m. By multiplication of the number of foot movements with the weight and the distance moved by the weight, the stress is given in kpm. We constructed a holding device for the ergometer so that the patient could put stress on his leg while lying in a supine position on the angiography table. With each patient we stressed the leg which showed the most marked symptoms.

5.3.3 Results

Table 8 shows the flow volumes in the arteria iliaca externa both before and after stress, as well as those on the unstressed opposite side. The mean flow volume at rest of all examined vessels is 446 ± 176 ml/min ($n=35$). Before exercise, the unstressed contralateral side showed a mean blood flow of 500 ± 136 ml/min ($n=16$), whereas the mean blood flow starting from rest of the stressed extremity was already lower at 393 ± 160 ml/min ($n=16$). The difference is significant in the associated t-test ($P=0.05$). After a mean ergometer strain of 323 kpm (range of 103–1200 kpm) the blood flow in the arteria iliaca externa rises markedly on the stressed side to 787 ± 343 ml/min (related t-test $P=0.001$), while the blood flow on the unstressed side remains constant at a mean value of 511 ± 176 ml/min. The mean flow rise on the stressed side was 120%.

5.3.4 Discussion

Although the blood flow in the arteria iliaca externa in this group of patients with ASO was measured after a single untriggered CM injection and not with the real-time sampling method, we regard the presentation of our results as justified for the following reasons:

Even if one considers the measurement of blood flow in our ASO patients by only one CM bolus as subject to greater inaccuracy than the twice-determined measurements from the real-time sampling method, it is still possible to demonstrate with our results the validity of videodensitometric flow measurements. *Itzchak* also measured the blood flow in the arteria iliaca externa densitometrically, with an untriggered CM bolus, in patients with ASO. We therefore have the same conditions, permitting a comparison of results. *Itzchak* states for his ASO patient

Table 8. Results of videodensitometric blood flow measurements in the arteria iliaca externa in patients suffering from arteriosclerosis obliterans

No.	Sex	Age	Side	r (mm)	Before stress V (ml/min)	After stress V (ml/min)	Stress (kpm)	Diff. (%)
1.	M	69	L.	2.5	684	681		0
			R.	2.5	123	569	231	362
2.	M	70	R.	3.7	549	516	240	−6
3.	M	60	R.	2.7	614	851	234	38
4.	F	67	R.	4.1	529	731	103	38
			L.	4.1	614	475		−22
5.	M	62	R.	3.1	225	207		−8
			L.	3.3	160	373	1005	133
6.	M	65	R.	4.2	375	502		33
			L.	4.1	651	1137	1200	74
7.	M	63	R.	2.5	393	498		26
			L.	2.4	427	1708	810	300
8.	M	75	R.	3.6	664	542		−8
			L.	3.5	293	605	180	106
9.	M	76	R.	3.0	410	644	198	57
			L.	3.1	792	500		−36
10.	M	66	R.	2.8	396	532		34
			L.	2.8	169	591	184	294
11.	M	62	R.	3.5	272	729	232	268
			L.	3.4	249	298		19
12.	M	43	R.	4.1	519	579		11
			L.	3.6	207	383	381	88
13.	M	49	R.	3.4	756	756		0
			L.	3.4	533	616	150	15
14.	M	63	R.	3.1	328	349		6
			L.	3.0	360	700	231	94
15.	M	53	R.	3.6	481	516		7
			L.	3.6	505	725	675	43
16.	M	63	R.	3.1	503	487		−3
			L.	3.0	481	699	195	45
17.	M	62	R.	3.2	366	1326	150	262
18.	M	77	R.	4.2	505	581		15
			L.	4.2	528	1057	165	100
19.	M	63	R.	2.9	692	616		−10
			L.	3.3	297	344	200	17

r, radius of arteria iliaca externa; Diff., difference between the measurements before and after stress

group that the mean flow volume in the arteria iliaca externa was 366±64 ml/min (n=21); we determined a somewhat higher flow of 446±176 ml/min (n=35). The deviation may result from a systematic error in the measurements of the vessel radius: the mean vessel radius in our group is larger (0.35±0.06 mm) than in Itzchak's group (0.31±0.05 mm).

We were able to prove with a group of 19 patients that the extremity with symptoms showing a higher degree of ASO also has a lower blood flow than the less affected opposite side. No similar investigation for comparison has been traced in the literature. We were also able to demonstrate that after stress the blood flow in the arteria iliaca externa rises significantly.

On account of the above-mentioned limitations in the accuracy of the measuring method, we dispensed with relating our measurements to the severity of ASO. Suffice it to state that under the given measuring parameters, the principal changes in the flow volumes of the arteria iliaca externa under stress in the lower extremity can be measured with videodensitometry. Further clinical studies should be conducted only with the ECG-triggered real-time sampling method. Starting with these basic methodical studies we regard it as sensible, without major additional intervention in the course of angiography, to measure the global blood flow under stress not only in the arteria iliaca externa, but also in the femoral arteries and the arteries of the lower leg. Information could be gained from these measurements on flow distributions in the stenosed arteries and collateral vessels, from which decisions for differential therapy may be deduced. For instance, it is often not clear to what extent a stenosis influences the hemodynamics, and whether therefore transluminal catheter dilation is indicated. Immediately after a dilatation of the stenosis one could without difficulty quantify a possible gain in blood flow. The chances of success of additional vascular surgery could then be judged with greater certainty.

6 Summary

The methods of angiography which are regularly used in clinical radiology allow an evaluation of peripheral vascular systems only from a morphological standpoint. X-ray videodensitometry, on the other hand, enables determination of blood flow volumes over defined vessel segments in the course of angiographic examinations, through a dynamic registration of changes in contrast medium (CM) density.

Wider clinical application of this method has so far been hindered by the cumbersome techniques and the imprecision of the measurements. In order to eliminate the first drawback, we developed a reasonably priced and easily handled analysis unit in the form of a personal computer for videodensitometrically measured CM density curves. The available mathematical calculation methods were cross-correlation and the standard and modified line-of-gravity methods.

Further research aimed to shed light on the measurement imprecisions inherent in the methods used. Measurements of calibration enabled us to ascertain that the X-ray equipment used behaved to a very large extent as a linear transfer system, and therefore could not be responsible for major measurement inaccuracies. On a circulation model with a continuous blood flow, we compared the conformity of videodensitometrically measured flow volumes with volumetrically given flow volumes. With the help of all three methods of calculation, an excellent coincidence of densitometrically measured and volumetrically given flow volumes could be demonstrated. It further emerged that the influence of the amount of CM injected on the accuracy of measurements is only minimal.

In further research, we examined with a circulation model the systematic influence of a pulsating flow on the accuracy of videodensitometric through-flow measurements. By way of cycle-phase-triggered injection of the contrast media, we were able to show a considerable over- and underestimation of densitometrically determined flow volumes at greater volumes and higher flow amplitudes, depending on the points of injection. At small flow volumes and low flow amplitudes, the videodensitometrically determined flow volumes showed no dependence on the phase position of the points of injection. The real-time sampling method recommended by *Vanselow* et al. for the determination of pulsating velocities was modified such that the mean value of the flow volumes of the CM boli injected at systolic and diastolic intervals was calculated by the line-of-gravity method. The mean value of both flow volumes showed a markedly higher correlation to the given flow than that achieved from a single bolus injection.

If one calculates the mean values of the flow volumes taken at points of injection spread over three or four pulse phases, then the real flow is increasingly overestimated. In clinical uses of videodensitometric flow measurements, one should therefore consider the influence of the pulsating flow and detect possible differences in measurements by using two ECG-triggered CM injections. In this way the real blood flow, in the sense of the real-time sampling method, is determined at great flow volumes or high flow amplitudes. If, however, small flow volumes or low flow amplitudes exist, then the real blood flow is measured on the principle of a simple double measurement.

In a comparison of the mathematical methods of analysis, it emerged that there is no ideal method of calculation. With the line-of-gravity method as modified by us, one can estimate the influence of sedimentation of CM at the end of a CM density curve. The cross-correlation analysis produces greater deviation from the real through-flow value for strongly pulsating flows than the line-of-gravity method, although its values are more reproducible.

The influence of pulsating blood flow on the reproducibility of videodensitometric through-flow measurements was investigated in 17 pelvic vessels in 13 patients. In the course of angiography two ECG-triggered CM boli were injected into the arteria iliaca externa at systolic and diastolic points. Analysis of the CM density curves was by the line-of-gravity method and cross-correlation.

The flow volumes determined at systolic injection points were contrasted with those at diastolic injection points. In agreement with the results from the pulsating flow models for low mean flow values at rest we found very high correlation coefficients and no systematic deviations between the two flow volumes. Here we found somewhat better correlation and lower estimated flow values with analysis by cross-correlation than with the line-of-gravity method. Since with low flow values at rest, the densitometrically determined flow volumes are not dependent on the pulsation of the blood flow, the estimation after phase-dependent ECG-triggered CM injections takes the form of a double measurement. With normal patients, whose mean blood flow at rest showed relatively high flow values, we measured a considerable difference between volumes at systolic and at diastolic injection times. In such cases the described phase-dependent CM injection has the advantage of producing, after two measurements, the mean blood flow according to the quasi-real-time sampling method.

In a further clinical study we demonstrated the practical application of videodensitometric flow measurements under the conditions of work hyperemia in a lower extremity, i.e., in the arteria iliaca externa. The measurements of flow at rest in patients with arteriosclerosis obliterans (ASO) showed good conformity with the measurements by another group of authors. The flow through the arteria iliaca externa was significantly smaller in the extremity with marked symptoms of ASO than on the other side. The mean blood flow in the arteria iliaca externa rose significantly after performance of ischemic leg exercise on an ergometer.

References

Borgnis F, Frutiger P (1969) An improved ultrasonic flowmeter. Cardiologia 54: 193
Brennecke R, Bürsch J, Heintzen PH (1978) Improvements in videodensitometry systems for cardiovascular studies. In: Heintzen PH, Bürsch J (eds) Roentgen-Video-Techniques. Thieme, Stuttgart, p 12
Brennecke R, Hahne HJ, Bürsch JH, Heintzen PH (1983) Digital videodensitometry: Some approaches to radiographic image restoration and analysis. In: Heuck FHW (ed) Radiological functional analysis of the vascular system. Springer, Berlin Heidelberg New York Tokyo
Bürsch J, Johs R, Heintzen PH (1969) Untersuchungen zur Gültigkeit des Lambert-Beerschen Gesetzes bei röntgenologischen Kontrastmittelmessungen. Fortschr Röntgenstr 112:259
Bürsch J, Kirbach H, Schnürer C, Heintzen PH (1971) Accuracy of videodensitometric flow measurement. In: Heintzen PH (ed) Roentgen-Cine- a. Videodensitometrie. Thieme, Stuttgart, p 119
Bürsch JH, Hahne HJ, Brennecke R, Grönemmeier D, Heintzen PH (1981) Assessment of arterial blood flow measurement by digital angiography. Radiology 141:39
Decker D, Roth FJ, Epple E, Allenberg JR (1973) Meßabweichungen der Röntgen-Cine-Densitometrie, überprüft an Modellabläufen. Biomed Technik 18: 133
Dedichen H, Kordt KF (1974) Blood flow in normal human ileo-femoral arteries studied with electromagnetic technique. Acta Chir Scand 140:371
Femor U, Huber H, Neuhaus KL, Schmiel FK, Spiller P (1979) Measurement of flow velocity in the model circulation by videodensitometry. Z Kardiol 73:361
Ganz V, Hlavoa A, Fronek A, Linhart J (1964) Measurement of blood flow in the femoral artery in man at rest and during exercise by local thermodilution. Circulation 30:86–93
Heuck F (1973) Densitometrie in der Radiologie. Thieme, Stuttgart
Heuck F (1983) Roentgen cinedensitometry of blood circulation. In: Heuck F (ed) Radiological functional analysis of the vascular system. Springer, Berlin Heidelberg New York Tokyo
Heuck F, Vanselow K, Deininger HK (1975) Neue Grundlagen und Theorien zur Verbesserung der Angio-Cine-Densitometrie. Fortschr Röntgenstr 123, 6:567–570
Heintzen PH (1971) Usefulness and limitation of conventional X-ray equipment for roentgendensitometric studies. In: Heintzen PH (ed) Roentgen-Cine- a. Videodensitometrie. Thieme, Stuttgart, p 1
Heintzen PH, Bürsch JH (1978) Roentgen-videotechniques. Thieme, Stuttgart
Heintzen P, Osypka P, Bürsch J (1969) New technique for functional studies in radiology and cardiology. Ann Radiol (Paris) 12:425
Hilal SK (1966) Determination of the blood flow by a radiographic technique. AJR 96:896
Itzchak Y, Yerushalmi S, Deutsch V (1975 a) Blood flow measurement in the iliac arteries by an improved angiographic cinedensitometrie technique. Invest Radiol 10: 1–9
Itzchak Y, Modan M, Adar R, Deutsch V (1975 b) External iliac artery blood flow in patients with arteriosklerosis obliterans. AJR 125:459
Jorfeldt L, Wahren J (1971) Leg blood flow during exercise in man. Clin Sci 41:459
Lantz B, Strid KG (1973) Contrast formation in fluoroscopic videodensitometry. II. A Comparison between theoretically computed and experimentally measured contrast. Acta Radiol 14:625

Lissner J, Marhoff P (1968) Videodensitometrie, technische Grundlagen und klinische Anwendung als Fernsehkymographie. Fortschr Röntgenstr 108:79
Pannek H, Neuhaus KL, Schmiel FK, Spiller P (1978) Röntgenvideodensitometrische Flußmessungen in aortokoronaren Bypass-Gefäßen. Z Kardiol 67:787
Piroth HD, Schmidt HD, Georgi M, Brünner H, Günther R, Leeder H (1979) Bestimmung der Leberhämodynamik im Rahmen der Splenoportographie bei portaler Hypertension. Fortschr Röntgenstr 130:311
Rosen L, Silverman NR (1973) Videodensitometric measurements of blood flow using cross-correlation technique. Radiology 109:305
Rutishauser W (1969) Kreislaufanalyse mittels Röntgendensitometrie. Huber, Bern
Rutishauser W, Bussmann WD, Noseda G, Meier W, Wellauer J (1970) Blood flow measurement through single coronary arteries by roentgen densitometry. I. A. Comparison of flow measured by a radiologic technique applicable in the intact organism and by electromagnetic flowmeter. AJR 109:12
Vanselow K, Heuck F, Deininger HK (1975) Neue Grundlagen und Theorien zur Verbesserung der Angio-Cine-Densitometrie. Fortschr Röntgenstr 123:468
Wood EH, Sturm RE, Sanders JJ (1964) Data processing in cardiovascular physiology with particular reference to roentgen videodensitometry. Mayo Clin Proc 39:849–865

Frontiers in European Radiology

Editors-in-Chief:
A. L. Baert, E. Boijsen, W. A. Fuchs, F. H. W. Heuck

Volume 3

1984. 80 figures in 143 separate illustrations. III, 136 pages. ISBN 3-540-11446-7

Contents: *C. Muhr, K. Bergström:* Modern Evaluation of the Sella Turcica. – *E. Starck, P. Harth, J. Kollath, H. E. Riemann, S. Tuengerthal, M. Walter:* Clinical Experience with Digital Subtraction Angiography. – *D. Claus:* Brain Ultrasonography in the Infant: A Review. – *P. Suetens, A. L. Baert, J. Gybels, S. Haegemans, P. Jansen, A. Oosterlinck, G. Wilms:* An Integrated 3-D Image of Cerebral Blood Vessels and CT View of Tumor. – *W. S. Rau, G. Renz, A. Tassinari-Renz, H. Friedburg, U. N. Riede, W. Wenz:* Pulmonary Edema and Shock Lung: Roentgenographic Observations on Pathologic Fine Structure of the Lung.

Volume 2

1982. 70 figures in 84 separate illustrations. V, 103 pages. ISBN 3-540-11349-5

Contents: *W. Loeffler:* NMR as an Imaging Method. – *R. E. Steiner, G. M. Bydder:* Initial Clinical Experience with NMR Imaging. – *F. W. Smith:* NMR Imaging of the Liver and Kidney. – *P. Marhoff, M. Pfeiler:* Digital Fluorography. – *M. P. Capp, S. Nudelman, D. Fisher, T. W. Ovitt, G. D. Pond, M. M. Frost, H. Roehrig, J. Seeger, D. Oimette:* Digital Radiography. – *A. B. Crummy, C. A. Mistretta:* Digital Subtraction Arteriography (DSA). – *T. F. Meaney, M. A. Weinstein, E. Buonocore, J. H. Gallagher:* Digital Subtraction Angiography: Cleveland Clinic Experience.

Volume 1

1982. 113 figures in 187 separate illustrations. V, 170 pages. ISBN 3-540-10753-3

Contents: *I. Fernström, B. Johansson:* Percutaneos Extraction of Renal Calculi. – *R. Günther, P. Alken:* Percutaneous Nephropyelostomy and Endo-Urological Manipulations. – *R. Pasariello, G. P. Feltrin, D. Miotto, S. Pedrazzoli, P. Rossi, G. Simonetti:* Transhepatic Portal Catheterization with Pancreatic Venous Sampling Versus Angiography in the Localization of Pancreatic Functioning Tumors. – *G. M. Kauffmann, G. Richter, J. Rassweiler, R. Rohrbach:* New Topics in Embolization. Effects of Central, Peripheral or Capillary Occlusion Type in Animal Models Simulating Tumor Embolization. – *F. Brunelle:* Electric Transcatheter Vascular Obliteration: Electrothrombosis. Electrolysis or Electrocoagulation. – *V. Hegedüs, O. Winding, J. Grønvall, P. Faarup:* Manifacturing-Derived Impurities in Angiography. – *K.-H. Hübener:* Digital Radiography Using a Computed Tomography Instrument.

Springer-Verlag
Berlin
Heidelberg
New York
Tokyo

MIX
Papier aus verantwortungsvollen Quellen
Paper from responsible sources
FSC® C105338

If you have any concerns about our products,
you can contact us on
ProductSafety@springernature.com

In case Publisher is established outside the EU,
the EU authorized representative is:
Springer Nature Customer Service Center GmbH
Europaplatz 3, 69115 Heidelberg, Germany

Printed by Libri Plureos GmbH
in Hamburg, Germany